Eczema

Itchin' For A Cure

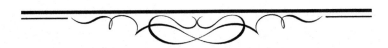

A little about the Author: Suzy Cohen, RPh

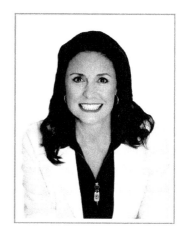

Hi there! I'm a conventionally trained pharmacist on a mission. Several specialties include drug side effects, thyroid disease, Lyme disease, neurological disorders and diabetes. In June 2014, I hosted an online, worldwide broadcast called The Thyroid Summit, *www.thethyroidsummit.com*

As a graduate of the University of Florida, I've been a licensed pharmacist since 1989. Because I believe that people should consider all their health options, not just medications, I've been studying Functional Medicine for almost two decades. I pride myself in thinking "outside the pill." And I do a lot of radio, TV, and other media to raise awareness for consumers about natural medicine. You can watch my television episodes with Dr. Oz and Dr. Mercola if you want to, go to my website *suzycohen.com* and click "media."

Since 1999, I have written a syndicated column called "Dear Pharmacist" that appears in newspapers nationwide.

Those columns are archived at my site and you can use the search box to read what I've written on various health topics.

I've authored many books, several went to #1 on Amazon in their category and I have them in various languages. Everything I write and offer you is the culmination of many years of intensive study, an educational track that I must pay thousands of dollars each year to obtain. The benefit of this tireless research and medical study is always given back to you.

Interested in more of my work? I have books to help you with all kinds of health concerns. These are my pride and joy. When you buy a book, you support my ability to research and write more articles and books. I really prefer doing this because in the grander scheme, it feels good to help. I like helping you this way so much more than dispensing drugs every day. Thank you!

Here are some of my other books, all available on Amazon:

Drug Muggers: Which Medications are Robbing Your Body of Essential Nutrients and How to Restore Them

Thyroid Healthy: Lose Weight, Look Beautiful and Live the Life You Imagine

The 24-Hour Pharmacist: Advice, Options and Amazing Cures from America's Most Trusted Pharmacist

Diabetes Without Drugs: The 5-Step Program to Control Blood Sugar Naturally and Prevent Diabetes Complications

Headache Free: Relieve Migraines, Tension, Cluster, Menstrual and Lyme Headaches

Understanding Pancreatitis: Vitamins, Teas and Herbal Remedies

Please be aware…

This book is not intended to treat, cure, or diagnose your condition. Your condition may require different treatments than those listed here. Please discuss any changes to your healthcare regimen with your physician and get approval before beginning (or discontinuing) any type of drug therapy, medication, or dietary supplement. As with any book that applies to health, individual safety must be the top priority. So please be advised that my recommended nutrients and nutrient dosages are meant as general guidelines, not gospel. They are not right for everyone. The information in this book is not intended as any kind of treatment. It's merely educational, for you to learn about various options that you should discuss with your doctor. Follow your instincts and always comply with your physician's advice. It's good to get second (and third) opinion when dealing with complex health conditions.

© 2012-2015 by DPI, Dear Pharmacist, Inc.
All rights reserved, including the right of reproduction in whole or part. To gain approval or information about reprinting sections, please write:
info@suzycohen.com
Cover design by Melissa Shanley Photography

Table of Contents

Introduction	Getting Started
Chapter 1	Eating Bugs is Good For You
Chapter 2	Metal Allergies Are Sometimes the Offender
Chapter 3	Food Sensitivity Testing
Chapter 4	The Power of Transfer Factor
Chapter 5	Skin-Soothing Supplements and Other Stuff!
Chapter 6	Fungus is Among Us
Chapter 7	Itchin' for A Cure- Avoiding Dry Skin
Chapter 8	Could It Be Your Medicine?
Chapter 9	Eczema Be Gone!
Chapter 10	Problem Genes?
Chapter 11	Nitty Gritty Stuff: Th1 vs. Th2 Immunity
Chapter 12	Dyshidrotic Eczema
Chapter 13	Castor Oil is a Comfy Alternative to Pain Medications
Chapter 14	Iodine: One Amazing Mineral
Chapter 15	Antihistamines to the Rescue
Chapter 16	My Review of Popular Skin Creams and Potions

Chapter 17	What if Your Addicted to Your Steroid?
Chapter 18	Looking at Light Therapy (Phototherapy)
Chapter 19	Acupuncture Can Help
Chapter 20	What Should You Wear?
Chapter 21	Dos and Don'ts
Bonus Section	Friends Helping Friends

Appendix 1- List of Topical Steroids

Getting Started!

No matter what part of your body is affected, the itching almost never stops. Whether all over your body or confined to your hands, if you have eczema, you're contending with an unsightly rash that you'd like to banish from your life forever. You not only want it healed, you don't want to see it, feel it or experience it ever again.

The disorder usually begins with something inside of you that malfunctions, whether it's a hyper-responsive immune reaction to food or a metal allergy, but regardless of that the tell-tale sign is a rash. And what a persistent and pesky rash it is! The skin dries out and becomes thickened or scaly; and the color may lighten or darken. In infants an oozing, crusty rash usually appears on the face, the scalp, or the bottom (although the rash can appear anywhere).

If you have eczema, you've likely spent thousands of dollars dealing with it, and you've paid dearly in other ways as well--with lack of comfort, not to mention normalcy. You don't need me to go on about how awful it is.

You totally get the picture, and would prefer that I focus on the cure, rather than the symptoms and appearance.

I'm not going to go into much detail about the causes of eczema. Honestly, the exact cause is not known yet, but there are lots of theories. The most solid one has to do with immune dysfunction, which I'll explain later. Most of this book will deal simply with helpful, healing information, about things you can avoid, supplements you can take, and topical creams and lotions that bring blessed relief.

I know how much you yearn for a cure for your condition, and to experience total comfort in your skin, once and for all. Be aware more than 30 million Americans have eczema, according to the National Eczema Association. I genuinely hope that you find something in my book to help you put an end to this condition once and for all. My goal in writing this book is to help you:

* Get rid of eczema without using medication

* Stop the itching

* Improve skin texture (reduce leather-like areas, called lichenification)

* Eliminate dry, cracked skin

* Ease the pain and blisters

* Avoid or get off prescription steroids creams

Sound good to you? Some people have asked me why I'm writing a book about eczema, when I don't have it myself. The answer is simple. I research all kinds of topics all day long. I've written books about other conditions that I don't have. I am in service to you. I started researching eczema very intensively in order to help a close friend that was experiencing a stubborn eczema flare. Aside from that, I've noticed an increasing frequency of questions about eczema on my Facebook page and website, so it was clear that many people needed help because the other books on the market weren't curing them, or providing enough relief.

The questions I received through email, and over face book were always the same desperate plea for help, for anything that would bring acute relief or a cure from the unsightly lesions and discomfort. Gosh, if you can't be comfortable in your own skin, how can you be comfortable? I thought to myself there has to be a better way than what you are doing now. I set out to find out as much as I could, and you are holding the result.

Below is the original question directed to my newspaper column that prompted some of my initial research:

Dear Suzy,

I have eczema on my right hand now, and I get episodic flares on both hands, which I am unable to attribute to anything in particular. It's very stubborn even though I've eliminated all dairy, grains and gluten. Any other suggestions?

--J.C., Boulder, Colorado

The answer to this question printed in newspapers nationwide, but was only a few paragraphs long, so what you are about to read is the full response which I have turned into a little book.

Chapter 1
Eating Bugs is Good for You

Most people think of eczema as an external skin problem and don't realize that what they eat strongly impacts how their skin reacts. Eczema affects people of all races, age, and gender. While it may be unsightly and uncomfortable at times, it is not contagious. So to be gluten, dairy and grain free is a good start, but in "J.C.'s" case it wasn't enough to completely clear the eczema from her hands where it would periodically flare. This means to me that there is something she is touching, or something else that she is eating that causes this, or something she is NOT doing for her immune system (which begins in the GI tract)... and on that note, I'm thinking of probiotics as a simple, inexpensive plan of action for her. And YOU too.

Think I'm crazy? Persistent eczema could absolutely be tied to poor probiotic status. Honestly, it could be as simple as improving gut flora. A study just published in *Clinical and Experimental Allergy* found that the strain *Lactobacillus rhamnosus* GG is particularly protective against eczema. Other studies concur.

This particular strain is sold by brand name Culturelle and there's a similar type called Del-Immune V. If you are avoiding dairy, be sure to purchase the Culturelle "Dairy-free" version. This would be my recommendation for you anyway because many people are sensitive to dairy and don't even know it. For general health, combine these products with a core probiotic that provides other healthy micro-organisms such as Dr. Ohhira's Probiotic, New Chapter's All-Flora, or Kyodophilus, or whatever your favorite is. My point here is that it's okay to combine the *L. rhamnosus* with another blend that you take every day. And yes, you do want to be on probiotics every single day.

We now know that many of the benefits to taking probiotics diminish about 2 weeks after stopping supplementation, so taking them daily is the best way to capitalize on the immune-modulating effects they provide. That's why they help with eczema.

In 2010, a study was published in *Pediatric Allergy and Immunology* to elucidate whether or not there was a preventative effect of probiotics on the development of eczema (atopic dermatitis), in particular infants at high risk.

This trial was good, meaning it qualified as randomized, double-blind and placebo-controlled. The researchers took 112 pregnant women who had a family history of allergic disease such as this, and gave half the ladies a probiotic supplement containing micro-organism strains such as Bifidobacterium bifidum, Lactobacillus acidophilus and others. The half of the group received a dud pill. They were given the probiotics (or the placebo dud pills) beginining 4-8 weeks prior to deliver and continued taking them for 6 months after delivery. Infants were breast-fed during the first 3 months, and months 4-6 were allowed formula. The prevalence of eczema in the group whose mom received probiotics was significantly lower than the placebo group. The researchers concluded "Prenatal and postnatal supplementation with a mixture of B. bifidum BGN4, B. lactis AD011, and L. acidophilus AD031 is an effective approach in preventing the development of eczema in infants at high risk of allergy during the first year of life." Simply put, eating bugs is good for you!

Not all the studies agree about using probiotics for skin problems. But while researchers debate the evidence, you might continue scratching yourself to death!

Why not give probiotics a try and see if they work for you? Probiotics are very safe, inexpensive, and fundamental for a healthy immune response.

Results are immediate, meaning that after suffering for many years, you could experience a dramatic improvement in your condition after taking probiotics for only a few weeks. Let's assume you are gluten, dairy and grain free, AND your probiotic supplement is high-quality. And you've tried taking probiotics and stayed committed to your clean diet for 2 months and you're still miserable. Then what?

Chapter 2
Metal Allergies Are Sometimes the Offender

This may shock you but some people react to metals that contain nickel, and nickel is all over the place--in coins, necklaces, eyeglasses, watches, and rings, for example. I'm serious, especially about the coins. There's even a new study out published in the July 2012 issue of *Contact Dermatitis* that is called "Coin exposure may cause allergic dermatitis."

The article contains this overview of problems with the element nickel found in coins: "For protection of the health of consumers, cashiers, and other workers who handle coins, it is suggested that coins without nickel release should be used as a substitute for the high nickel-releasing coins currently in widespread use. The key risk factor in this situation is the ability of metal alloys in coins to release nickel and contaminate the skin after repeated contact from coin handling."

We knew about this problem as far back as 1991, when a case report was published in the August issue of the *Journal of the American Academy of Dermatology* featuring a 48-year-old cashier with hand eczema and a genuine nickel allergy. Eczema is actually common in cashiers. It would make me think twice about counting out exact change if I happen to have hand eczema, as I do this frequently, much to the annoyance of people standing in line behind me. I should tell you that hand eczema is sometimes termed "dyshidrotic eczema" and there's a section on this later on in my book. Everything that applies to hand eczema applies to the full-body sort which is sometimes called atopic eczema. Don't worry about the names, the point here is that metals can be a problem for many people with skin conditions.

If you are one of these folks, it's easy to remedy. I suggest that you remove all your jewelry and not touch coins for a few weeks. Definitely avoid white gold and costume jewelry. Even 10 and 14k gold can trigger you, so wear only 18-24K gold if you must.

I found a product that tests for nickel in your items, so your skin doesn't have to. It's called "The Nickel Solution Kit" by Athena Allergy. You can also buy a little bottle of "Nickel Guard" from that company and paint it on your glasses or your jewelry to stop the rash you would normally get from these items. I asked my friend to vouch for the efficacy of Nickel Guard so she purchased it off their site and when we went I saw her next she was wearing earrings. I said how are you wearing earrings now? She said the "Nickel Guard" was working, she had painted it on the back of her diamond earring studs and could now wear them. So while this is just one testimony, it's a big deal to me because my friend is highly (repeat highly) sensitive to nickel, and the product worked for her. You can try it too, and let me know what your response is. To learn more about the Nickel Solution Kit or Nickel Guard, visit Athena's website: www.AthenaAllergy.com

Just FYI, there are two homeopathic medications that I know of. The first one is called Psorizide Forte and supposedly desensitizes you to nickel by giving you homeopathic nickel. That is so super cool to me, assuming it really works. The ingredients are:

Fumaric Acid- It inhibits keratinocyte proliferation, or basically blocks the skin cells from growing wildly and in excess.

Potassium Bromide- A mineral, given in homeopathic form that is given in combination with nickel. In the gut, this molecule breaks down into it's two ions. As an aside, I found this interesting, the compound "potassium bromide" been studied in much higher doses (in Germany) for it's anti-convulsant effect but it's not approved for use in the United States.

Nickel sulphate- Yes, nickel, the same nickel I just told you that you might be allergic to but it's a homeopathic version so you have to think of it as a molecule that has the essence of nickel. The point of it being here is to present a form of nickel to your body in teeny-tiny (homeopathic) doses so that you become desensitized to it.

Your doctor must prescribe the drug Psorizide Forte. It is indicated for the treatment of contact dermatitis, allergies to nickel (metals and jewelry), dyshidrotic hand/foot eczema and mild to severe eczema or psoriasis. Plymouth Pharmaceuticals makes it.

I mentioned there was a second medication available that works just as well as this one, if not better.

It's called Eczemol and it's also made by Plymouth Pharmaceuticals. The ingredients are slightly different. This product is dosed 300mg and 1 tablet is taken once daily. The website boasts that this is safe for young children and the tablets dissolve easily. The ingredients in Eczemol include two of the three ingredients in their other product listed above (Psorizide Forte), and those are nickel sulfate and fumaric acid. Instead of the potassium bromide, they put in homeopathic sulfur. I like this because sulfur is a natural mineral to the human body. Sulfur is radically different than "sulfa" which refers to a drug component that many people are allergic to. Sulfur and sulfa are as different as an elephant and a bird.

I love sulfur in this product because it is giving you a natural anti-fungal, anti-bacterial, anti-viral and anti-parasitic properties. Not only that, but sulfur promotes skin health in a variety of ways. If I'm picking for you, I buy Eczemol, and try that one first, over the Psorizide Forte, but this is up to you. **Plymouth Pharmaceuticals** has information about both products that I've mentioned here. You can't buy it at the website, you have to ask your physician to prescribe it. That's because it's a prescription drug as bizarre as that sounds (because it's homeopathic so it SHOULD be over-the-counter) but hey I don't make these rules.

What Are You Touching?

My friend would always get a consistent rash on her right hand, to go with the flares on other parts of her body and as I mentioned she had a clean diet, a high-quality probiotic and she insisted she was not touching metal. When I thought about it long enough, I realized she was touching metal, lots of it! Every day, for hours all day long! It was her laptop, she types on it as part of her job, and wouldn't you know it, her palms were paying the price for touching the metal all day long as she typed!

You can call me Nancy Drew if you'd like, but some of you are touching things that you don't even realize and if you are highly sensitive to nickel, aluminum or any other metal, it's going to trigger a flare. For my friend, the problem was solved when she bought yoga gloves by Gaiam (with the holes cut off the fingers) and she was able to type all day with no more flares. Yay!

You could use cotton gloves purchased from a department store if you want them to be made of this particular fabric, and just cut your own finger holes to type.

If you have eczema, particularly hand eczema (dyshydrotic) take a minute and ask yourself the following questions:

1. Do I use a metallic pen that might contain nickel?

2. Do I hold my cell phone in that hand, and/or does it have a case that might be triggering the rash?

3. Do I hold my sweetie's hand so that my own skin is touching his jewelry? (If so try holding his or her other hand instead. Or ask your beloved to remove hand jewelry so it doesn't come into contact with you.)

4. Do I hold the gear shift on my car with my right hand? Perhaps it contains nickel or other metals that trigger this reaction?

5. Is there metal on the dog leash that I use to walk my dog?

6. Am I a coin user? Some people like to count out exact change to pay for stuff.

7. Do I handle stainless steel pots by their handles? (You can buy cloth or rubber coverings at department stores and kitchen stores, so that your hand doesn't have to touch the handles directly. I personally would recommend switching from stainless, because you're still ingesting nickel, even though you're not touching it. Perhaps cast iron, nano ceramic cookware, or glassware (for baking) are better options. This is personal, but I would avoid aluminum or Teflon myself.

8. Do I type on a laptop where my palms graze a metal-containing surface?

Testing for Metal Allergy

It's actually quite easy to find out for sure whether you are allergic to metals. I hate to bring this up, but the problem is not limited to coins, jewelry, and kitchenware. And it's not limited to nickel either. Chronic exposure to a variety of metals in things like dental implants, restorations, vascular stents, and prosthesis could very well be the underlying cause for your skin problems and allergic reactions.

You can take a simple blood test, which will tell you whether or not you are suffering from side effects of metal exposures. It's called the MELISA test, and will help you sort out which metals your body can tolerate, and which it cannot. Visit www.melisa.org for more information. The test will indicate any sensitivity to a wide spectrum of metals such as gold, cobalt, chromium, palladium, titanium, tin, nickel, cadmium, phenyl mercury, and inorganic mercury. I recommend this type of metal allergy testing for people with eczema. It's also a good idea for anyone with of with autism, scoliosis, multiple sclerosis, chronic fatigue, fibromyalgia, or osteoporosis.

If you ask your physician to test you for metal sensitivity, more than likely he or she will suggest a skin test. That's okay as far as I'm concern, but I think a blood test is better because the lab will use your own lymphocytes (the immune cells found in your blood that hop to it and attack anything they perceive as a threat) to see how they react to various metals.

There are a variety of panels to choose from that most fit your lifestyle and exposures. The blood is incubated for a week, and then levels of reactivity are measured. With the MELISA test, a value over 3 indicates a positive reaction. The report is sent to your physician; and of course you can get a copy.

Neuroscience Labs, one of my favorite labs, offer a panel that checks you for hypersensitivity to 16 metals. Your doctor has to order this test for you, it's called The Melisa Metals I & II. Here's a list of the metals in this panel that they check you for: aluminum, cadmium, chromium, cobalt, copper, gold, lead, nickel, platinum, silver, thimerosal, titanium dioxide, inorganic mercury, ethylmercury, methylmercury, phenylmercury. You or your doctor can visit their website.
This lab also has other, less comprehensive, less expensive tests.)

Orthopedic Analysis is another company that offers metal allergy testing. The test is called "Metal-LTT Metal Allergy Testing." The "LTT" stands for "lymphocyte transformation test" and it measures the activity of immune cells that are exposed to suspected metal allergens, just like the test offered by MELISA. You can find more about this company at *www.orthopedicanalysis.com*

One more comment to spare you confusion. I've written and promoted various companies such as Doctors Data, Genova, or Metametrix (those last two labs recently merged together), for various heavy metal evaluations via tests that use urine. Tests such as these are for the purpose of determining what kinds of type of metals may be contaminating your body. These metals are literally stuck inside you and will spill out of you upon provocation with chelating agents. Those types of tests are wonderful, but to clarify, they are NOT at all what I'm suggesting here. The metal allergy test I'm recommending for people with eczema is intended to help you identify which metals you react to when you come into contact with them, not to see how much arsenic, lead, or mercury is inside of you. While that's interesting, I don't think it will help you determine the underlying cause of your skin condition.

Every now and then I hear from a reader that says their doctor wants to do a skin prick test or an intra-dermal injection to gauge reaction. *Um, can I just say no?* You see, in these tests the skin is pricked with a needle and a solution with the suspected allergen is put into you. The amount of antigen applied to you is teeny tiny, and the point is to see if there is a reaction on your skin. It helps to diagnose dermatitis and skin sensitivities. but I don't think it's as effective as the blood tests I'm recommending above. Also, who wants what they are allergic to put into them? Blood testing is more reliable. *Maybe it's just me, but I'd want to stay as far away as possible from what I was sensitive too, and would rather offer a sample of my blood for testing any day.*

Eat Less Metal and Other Trigger Foods
Don't freak out, but you might be eating large amounts of nickel. I think I just heard you say, "Huh?" It's true! Some foods actually contain small amounts of nickel, and it can trigger systemic contact dermatitis. I'd minimize or avoid dark chocolate. I feel bad saying that, truly I'm not an ogre, but pure cocoa powder has a nickel concentration of about 10 mcg/g. Dark chocolate is a little better but still high 2.6 mcg/g. And before you hate on me for telling you not to eat chocolate, let me just say that this is not a forever thing.

Once your immune system chills out and stops fighting with you (it could take a few weeks or months), you can add it back in, okay?!

I don't think chocolate is the cause of eczema; that's ludicrous. I just think it could be one trigger food because it's high in nickel, and often contains dairy. That's a whole other topic that you can research on your own. Other high nickel foods include mussels, licorice, soy beans, beans, chickpeas, oatmeal, and pretty much every nut there is.

Also, avoid canned foods if you're sensitive and switch from stainless steel cookware to cast iron. There are some experts that suggest eating foods high in vitamin C and iron, but the use of iron supplements is not recommended for people with heart disease or cancer. Cooking in cast iron pots should not pose a problem however, because the amount imparted during cooking is miniscule.

Chapter 3
Food Sensitivity Testing

You may also want to cut out all the common food allergens such as eggs, soy, wheat/gluten, dairy/casein, corn, tree nuts, shellfish (shrimp, crab, lobster), and anything boxed or processed for just 1 month and eat only natural nutritious foods and see what happens. If you get better, you can bring back one new food group at time, such as nuts. If the itch comes back then you will have connected the dots and you'll have a good handle on your personal trigger foods are.

You might also consider being tested to find out exactly which foods and spices you're sensitive to. One of the best companies for this is U.S. BioTek. Just so you know, the clinical relevance of food or inhalant specific antibody testing (like for IgA and IgG) is not technically established, so if you get a test result that is positive (meaning you have high IgA or IgG antibodies to a particular substance), it really represents exposure to a food or inhalant allergen. Exposure is different than allergy. As such test results must be evaluated by the health care provider who understands the limitations of these types of tests.

Nevertheless, I think the tests are a good way to see what your body creates antibodies to. You can eliminate those particular foods and see if you get better or not. You have nothing to lose.

Okay, if you are not too upset with me for telling you to cut out chocolate, read on because I have other important considerations.

Chapter 4
The Power of Transfer Factor

All of you have heard of colostrums, the milk produced from mother in the first few days after childbirth. It contains all kinds of important immune factors that are passed from or "transferred" from the mother to the child. Let's call those "Transfer Factors" like all the scientists do when conducting research. You can also buy the supplement called "Transfer Factor" at any health food store or online retailer. The molecules are derived from cow's milk or from egg yolk protein (not humans) when you buy the supplement. The point of mentioning this is to inform you that you can improve immune function and rebalance it with Transfer Factor supplements. They are particularly good for people with autoimmune disorders and allergic reactions such as eczema. They are more of an immune system balancer, and perhaps a stimulator.

Many people with allergy or sensitivity to milk wonder whether they can take Transfer Factor since the molecules are derived from milk.

It just depends; this supplement does not contain casein (the protein found in milk), so if that is your specific allergy then you are fine. But if you are sensitive to some other component in milk then you should consider taking only the egg yolk-derived supplements of Transfer Factor. The label will tell you whether the product is derived from milk or from egg yolks.

You should also be aware that Th1 dominant conditions, such as psoriasis, are not helped by Transfer Factor, and could actually be made worse. If you're wondering what "Th1 dominant" means, I will explain that shortly, in an upcoming section.
I only mention here because some of you with psoriasis sometimes take this product, and it might not be right for you.

Another way to get the immunoglobulins found in colostrum would be to consume whey protein. Again, it's best to avoid this option if you are sensitive to dairy products, but a high quality whey protein can supply your body with extra support for your immune system. In addition to immunoglobulins, whey provides other critical co-factors such as lactoferrin and alpha lactalbumin, which together help create the perfect recipe or metabolic environment for production of a potent antioxidant called glutathione. Glutathione supports liver health and reduces toxins in the body.

Chapter 5
Skin-Soothing Supplements and Other Stuff!

While we're on the topic of supplements, let me just go ahead and provide you with recommendations for a whole host of supplements and topical products that could bring relief.

Vitamin D. The fact is that a good portion of the population in this country does not get enough of this vitally important vitamin. The best way to tell if you fall short is to request a simple blood test from your doctor. Make sure your blood levels are above 50, preferably closer to 70. Ask your doctor for a 25(OH) vitamin D level test--the best indicator of blood levels. If your levels are low, I suggest taking Vitamin D3, purchased over-the-counter in dosages of about 5,000 daily for a month or two. Then you can retest, and move your dosage up or down from there. The most usable form of vitamin D is D3 (not D2 which is sold by prescription in the amount of 50,000 IU taken once a week). So read your label carefully and buy natural D3, which is sold at health food stores. For more information on vitamin D, visit www.vitamindcouncil.org

Essential Fatty Acids (EFAs). Abundant in fish oil, EFAs have been consistently shown to support skin health. In a double-blinded study published in *Lancet*, 18 people with psoriasis were given 10 fish oil capsules daily, so they were getting a lot of EFAs each day. The control group received a placebo containing nothing more than olive oil. The group taking fish oil capsules reported significant reductions in itching, redness. and the size of the skin lesions. None of the people in the control group improved during the three-month study.

While this study pertains to psoriasis, not eczema, I still know that EFAs benefit both groups of people. Why? Science has shown that people who suffer with eczema do have problems with fatty acid metabolism, they are usually missing an enzyme that normally changes certain dietary fats into the biochemicals that are needed for healthy skin. These people have more of what's called "cis-linoleic acid" and less of the desired gamma linoleic acid (GLA). There is essentially a defect in their ability to convert linoleic acid to GLA, which is the stuff you want. I'll spare you all the science here, but just know that fish oils and GLA supplements may do the trick for you.

If you're really up on your study of what causes inflammation—and many people who have eczema are, it's just possible that you'll want to email me the following question:

Suzy - You recommend GLA for eczema. Isn't GLA an omega-6 fatty acid that promotes inflammation? Wouldn't it be better to take omega-3s in the form of fish oils and skip the GLA?

So here's my response, so you don't have to email me now: It IS true that a high ratio of omega-6 to omega-3 fatty acids in a person's diet promotes inflammation by favoring synthesis of prostaglandins, which can be pro-inflammatory hormones. But the amount of GLA needed to treat eczema and other skin conditions (500 milligrams twice a day) is too small to affect that ratio significantly, especially if you are taking those fish oils I just recommended. I recommend taking a ratio of 4:1 of EPA and DHA to GLA. So for example if you are taking 2000 milligrams of EPA/DHA, then you need 500 milligrams of GLA.

GLA is a pretty cool fatty acid found in evening primrose oil, black currant oil, and borage oil. It's very hard to come by in the diet, even if you eat a healthy diet. It has specific nourishing effects on skin, hair, and nails that can't be accomplished by omega-3 fatty acids alone. That's why I recommend supplemental GLA for any allergic skin condition such as eczema.

There is a tremendous amount of research on EFAs and GLA. So if you want to know more, just google it. The bottom line is that eczema responds to healthy fats and that's my point. Taking these supplements is one of the most important things you can do to experience relief.

How much should you take? I suggest 2,000 to 4,000 mg total daily dose of omega 3 fish oils, which provide you with both EPA/DHA. You can work your way up to that. If you are sensitive, don't start that high all at once.

One of my new favorite fish oil supplements is made by Barleans. It's called Omega Swirl and I swear to you it's not fishy at all. It tastes like a creamy smoothy. It provides 1,500 mg EPA/DHA in each serving, and it's free of artificial sweeteners. It's an ultra high potency blend of fish oils that contains double the omega 3 potency of most other brands, and it tastes fruity. Oh wow, I promise you there is no nasty, oily texture. (Do I sound like a commercial? Sorry, they don't pay me to say this, lol). You don't have to swallow large capsules (yay!), and it comes in yummy flavors: Orange Cream, Key Lime, Mango Peach, and a few others. This product should be carried in most health food stores, and if it's not just ask them to order it. I pour this stuff over fresh organic strawberries, drink it straight, and put some in my smoothies and then think about when I can take my next dose... lol.

Other good brands of fish oil include those from Xymogen, Nordic Naturals, Nature Made, and Carlsons. Fish oils are what I recommend, not krill, not flax. Also, for the GLA component, I suggest about 500 mg taken twice daily with food, and you can work your way up to that too.

Lavender essential oil. You may know this best as an herbal tranquilizer, but one of its most incredible virtues is its skin-supportive features. Lavender is also known botanically as *Lavandula angustifolia*. Buy pure oil, sometimes you can even find it in a convenient roll-on bottle, and apply a few drops to those small patches of dry, itching, scaling areas. You don't have to dilute it, but you can if you want. Compounds in lavender reduce inflammation quite effectively, plus they have antiseptic, antimicrobial, and antifungal properties.

Tea Tree essential oil. This can be very healing, and it's simple. Because it's very strong, I'd recommend just putting about 3 to 5 drops in your bath. Tea tree acts as an astringent, and antifungal, and is known to benefit people with skin conditions of all sorts. Dessert Essence Tea Tree Oil Skin Ointment is a brand that comes highly recommended from an eczema sufferer, who she swears by this product. It contains various essential oils and herbal extracts that soothe dry, chapped skin on face and body. I think it can work especially well for dry scalp patches. If you wax your legs, armpits, or places where the sun don't shine, you might also like this product after the waxing treatment.

I recommend tea tree infused soap as well. This soap smells really good. Do be aware that pure essential oil of tea tree has a strong aroma. It's not unpleasant, just something that takes getting used to.

Betaine hydrochloride or TMG. This is a digestive acid, and people with chronic eczema are usually low in digestive acids. It's sold OTC but it's not for everyone. It may cause heartburn in some people. Ease into this supplement slowly. Take one with each meal, and if you do not get heartburn, try two with each meal, and so forth. Keep increasing until you get that familiar burn, then back off. If low acid is your problem, then your skin will clear up accordingly. Getting enough acid into your system can have dramatic health benefits, too numerous to include here. You should put in the word "betaine" at my website, in the search box, *suzycohen.com* and see what else I say about betaine. While we're on the subject of stomach acid, if you are currently taking acid blocking medications for reflux and GERD, you might want to take some time later on to read my other article at my website entitled "Dangerous Drug Mugging Effect by Acid Blockers."

Inositol. I'm on the fence about this one, but I want you to be armed with as much information as possible. So, here goes: Inositol powder does seem to help prevent eczema outbreaks. A dietary supplement sold at health food stores, inositol is a naturally occurring substance that is part of the phospholipids in animals. In plants, it is contained in phytic acid, which can bind iron, zinc, and calcium, so plant sources may deplete the body of these minerals.

Most experts believe that inositol is produced by gut bacteria. (There I go again, advocating a healthy gut, complete with probiotics.) Here's the thing; drinking coffee can deplete your stores of gut bacteria and thus also deplete your store of inositol. So restoring gut bacteria with probiotics, and possibly taking inositol for a few weeks may be part of the picture for you. It will help with cell membrane structure and skin integrity. But I would not recommend taking inositol supplements long term; there's no need since your body automatically makes what you need.

You may want to take it, however, if you drink coffee daily, or suffer with other problems related to inositol deficiency, such as constipation, hair loss, high cholesterol, nerve pain, or vision problems.

Inositol supplements are taken along with choline and B complex supplements for best absorption. Note that phytic acid in food is known to interfere with absorption of various minerals, like zinc and iron. It's best to take inositol at a different time than all other supplements, except for B vitamins.

Coconut. Drink coconut water, and buy coconut oil to cook with and to apply to your skin. Seriously, you can use it like you would any lotion. **Research is only now beginning to verify the strong health benefits of coconut oil.** In one study published in *Skin Pharmacology and Physiology*, scientists found that when virgin coconut oil is applied to a wound, it dramatically increases the rate at which wounds heal. Compounds tend to speed healing by stimulating collagen production and cell turn-over. Also, the process of forming new blood vessels improves in skin treated with virgin coconut oil.

Soap Matters

The kind of soap you use makes a huge difference. Avoid those with fragrances, phthalates and SLS. In fact, avoid commercial soaps altogether, especially the liquid scented ones that you pour onto a scrubby in the shower. I suggest avoid antibacterial soaps as well, as they are harsh and drying (not to mention the fact that they contribute to antibiotic resistance).

Soaps that contain glycerin are wonderful. Shea butter is also a helpful ingredient in soaps and lotions, as it is loaded with vitamins A, D, E, and F, all of which nourish skin. You may not have heard of vitamin F, and if that's the case, I'll tell you that it's basically made up of fatty acids and comes in two forms: omega 3 and omega-6; it's primarily role is to repair and create tissue in the body.

Castile soap is another good option. It's made with olive oil and will gently cleanse and moisturize you or your baby's delicate skin. Look for natural castile soap made with 100 percent olive oil, because some makers use other vegetable oils to make castile soap. Use either solid or liquid castile soap. Castile soap contains a large amount of vegetable glycerin and as you just learned, glycerin is soothing because it helps retain moisture.

If you need a nice hand soap for your bathroom, one that you can pump out, I've done the homework already. My two favorite ones are:

Kiss My Face Organic Grapefruit & Bergamot Self-Foaming Liquid. This one is in my bathroom right now. (Also comes in Lemon Ginger scent). Most self-foaming hand soaps contain propellants to create the instant foam. This one does not; the pump action happens without harsh chemical propellants. It contains flowers, herbs, and aloe, plus essential oils to clean your hands, no artificial colors, and no animal ingredients. (They make a bar soap made of pure olive oil too.) *www.kissmyface.com*

Pangea Organics Hand Soap Italian White Safe with Geranium & Yarrow. This is in my other bathroom right now. It contains coconut, jojoba and olive oil as the base with extracts of essential oils for natural antimicrobial effect. *www.pangeaorganics.com*

Both of these soaps are usually sold at places like Whole Foods or other health food stores. You will not find them at the local pharmacy or at your favorite big box store, so don't bother looking. You can buy them online at Amazon or other online retailers. I've provided the websites above for each company. By the way, both these companies offer other impressively clean and pure products that you might like as part of your total personal care arsenal.

It gets awkward sometimes...

Because well-meaning dermatologists recommend that you clean up is with Cetaphil, Aveeno, Olay or Dove bath bars, cleansers and soaps. Feh... I'm not excited with those, but for transparency, I'm not a dermatologist, just a nerdy pharmacist who has discovered her inner herbal gene! This is where I stand (*and I never want to stand between you and physician orders*), but those brands are just okay for people with psoriasis or eczema, in my opinion.

You see, even those supposedly gentle or "delicate" soaps as touted on their labels happen to contain ingredients that you might react to. Oftentimes, they are laden with ingredients that are not pronounceable (because they are synthetic), or they have sulfates, SLS, phthalates, or other hidden ingredients to go with the gentle ones. Sometimes, it's just an artificial dye or a preservative. You see, I feel that there are better soaps for people with super-sensitive, nagging skin problems. I've already discussed glycerin, and liquid castile. Elsewhere in this book, I mention seaweed-based soaps, powders for your bath as well as body and scalp treatments.

I mentioned tea tree essential oil earlier. Now I want to tell you about soaps containing tea tree oil (a.k.a. **melaleuca oil**). **Tea tree oil** is a natural antiseptic and antifungal essential oil. Many brands of soap contain tea tree oil; and you have to find those at your health food store. I like tea tree for eczema.

There's enough evidence for me to confidently recommend you try this essential oil and soaps that contain the oil. I found one such product on Amazon by Nubian Heritage. It's called Lemongrass and Tea Tree Soap. There's another type of Nubian Heritage soap called Nubian Raw Shea Butter Soap, which is also excellent for eczema,. It contains frankincense and smells a little more "manly," I'm told from one of my male readers.

Other soaps I recommend are those containing sulfur, such as Grisi's "Sulfur soap with lanolin." I found it at this link for about three U.S. dollars on Amazon

Sulfur is well known to help with eczema, psoriasis, and acne. Yet another soap I recommend is called **Kampuku Beauty Bar** by Dr. Ohhira (Essential Formula's Inc). This beauty bar is one I use every day in my shower, it's feels and works like soap and it contains a blend of probiotics that help restore healthy micro-organisms to your skin, and the friendly bacteria actually act as a natural humidifying agent. A lot goes into making this beauty bar. It takes them 5 years to make it, and even though many raw ingredients are used to create the soap (which you might think you are sensitive to, such as wild strawberry, Shiitaki mushroom, Chinese bayberry, apricot, brown seaweed, loquat, etc), I still think this soap is worth a try. The reason is that I've heard many remarkable stories from people who tried it with great success. You can buy Kampuku Beauty bars at health food stores (if they don't stock, just ask them to order it for you), or buy it yourself online.

If you follow my work, you already know that I like **Dr. Ohhira's Probiotic.** This is the company that makes this soap! I asked (and received) a coupon code that enables you to get a free sample of this beauty bar. It's a substantial sample; something you can truly use. It's free to you if you buy any of their products, for example, their Dr. Ohhira's Probiotics (which I do recommend and take myself), or their vegan essential fatty acid product Essential Living Oils. Anyway, the coupon code is "suzy12" and it gives you the free bar of Kampuku Soap, as well as free shipping, and the prices are already discounted as compared to other retailers.

And speaking of sulfur, did you know that the magnesium sulfate salts (better known as Epsom salts) provide a perfect version of sulfur for your skin to absorb? Epsom salts are carried by your local drugstore and they are a marvelous remedy for those suffering from skin ailments. Epsom salts break down in water and give your skin a soothing sulfur treatment. You put a 6 or 8 cups in a warm bath and it is an excellent gentle way to detox and soothe your skin. I buy 25 pound bags from Saltworks or other online stores, because I hate running out on a cold, snowy night.

Concerned about side effects of using a lot of salt in your bath? Don't be! The side effect of Epsom salts are wonderful! The side effect is that your sore and achy joints or bruises will feel better, so you will come out of your bath feeling regenerated inside and out. For an incredibly soothing bath, add some bentonite clay to the Epsom salts bath, and you'll feel silkier and softer when you get out.

One company actually produces my favorite bath salt with clay, already prepared. I am never ever without this bath salt in my house. It's made by Redmond Trading and they offer a variety of salts, but the one I recommend is Bath Salt Plus, because it has a high concentration of minerals that come from a sea bed dating back thousands of years, combined with natural clay. The addition of clay is why they call it "Plus." This combination is detoxifying and remineralizing to the body, There are two sizes of Redmond Bath Salt Plus. One costs about $9 and the other $20. I asked Redmond for a coupon for my readers, and was given one. If you go to checkout and put in my name "suzycohen" it will give you 15% off your entire order.

Just as an aside, if you spend more than $35 USD, you get free shipping. (However, you have to take into account the 15% discount, which may cause you to fall below the $35).

Seaweed to the Rescue

Some anecdotal evidence supports the use of seaweed-based personal care products to fight flaking and eczema concerns. One good company to check out is Seaweed Bath Company. The founder of this company, Adam Grossman, has dealt with psoriasis, a severe inflammatory skin condition just like eczema. This company makes shampoos, body washes, and soaps that might be soothing to your skin. One of their coolest products is **Wildly Natural Seaweed Argan Conditioner**, which combines the naturally nourishing and detoxifying properties of bladderwrack seaweed with soothing argan oil and other ingredients to gently moisturize your hair and scalp. Argan oil is something I recommend and that you'll read about later. They also offer Natural Seaweed Powder Baths, as well as natural seaweed body butters and bath wash. All their products are free of SLS, dyes, and parabens.

Chapter 6
Fungus Is Among Us

You can't talk about eczema without mentioning fungus or yeast. Yeast organisms can grow on the skin surface and, according to some experts, this may actually be the cause of eczema. I interviewed Doug Kaufmann, host of Know the Cause TV (*www.knowthecause.com*) and one of the nation's leading authorities on fungus. He's written 8 books on fungus including, *Fungus is a Cancer*. He wanted you to know this: *"After 6 years of clinical work in a large Dermatology clinic in Dallas, Texas, we were all convinced that eczema is an inside problem manifesting outside!"*

No doubt on my part, because as you know the skin is just a mere reflection of what is happening on the inside, and sometimes, it is the only way out a toxin has. So I persisted and asked Doug what some of the most effective treatments he saw used in the patients there, and he offered: *"Omega 3 fatty acids helped some patients, whereas the medication Nystatin helped others. Overwhelmingly however, since most of these sufferers crave carbohydrates, we were able to see remarkable changes just by changing their diets and putting them on what I today call the 'Phase One Diet'. The reduction in carbs and grains was very beneficial. This is why my diet (which does allow berries, grapefruit, and green apples by the way) was able to help patients seeking our help to obtain significant results. The medications and supplements were incidental to the major changes achieved by eliminating mold- and fungus-forming foods."*

Did you hear that? Mold! When Doug said "mold" to me, it opened up a can of worms and a major "Ah ha!," because I knew a lot of people in Florida who had asthma, allergies, and eczema.

When I think back on that, I wonder how much of it had to do with mold exposure. I've lived in Florida before, for a total of 35 years in fact, so I've seen my share of mold stains on walls and remember the smell of it on hot, humid days.

Thankfully I stayed far enough away from areas where it was flourishing, so it did not affect my health. But what if you do have to live in a humid area? What if you stack firewood in your home or out back... that's a great spot for mold formation. You could be unaware of the mold in your home because it is deeply hidden inside air vents, the damp basement (you can smell the musty mold, you know), or behind a wall that has been repainted and so on. Doug urged me to inform you that that mold can easily provoke eczema. Easily!

Mold organisms are among the most hazardous household substances for people with allergies and asthma. Is it the chicken or the egg? Does the mold trigger the asthma attacks and allergic reactions (such as eczema or hay fever) or does it invade your body because your immune system is weakened from the conditions above? Did you know that mold can cause health issues of every sort in people without eczema?

There are studies all over the Internet regarding particular fungi called Malassezia, which are closely tied to eczema and psoriasis. This was shown in the *Public Library of Science* June 2012 issue, which featured a study entitled, "Malassezia fungi are specialized to live on skin and associated with dandruff, eczema, and other skin diseases." This was echoed in another journal, *Clinical Microbiological Reviews*, when the authors discussed the well-known cushy relationship of this fungi to eczema.

More specifically, the authors state, "A close association between skin and Malassezia IgE binding allergens in atopic eczema has been shown, while laboratory data support a role in psoriasis exacerbations."

What they're saying is exactly what Doug is saying, that mold/fungus is eerily united, and eliminating the organisms could help you. Well, it certainly couldn't hurt!

Doug used to ask his patients this key question, *"Have you taken a vacation and do you frequently feel better when you travel?"* If the answer is yes to that question, you must always think of indoor mold as a probable cause until proven otherwise! Just FYI, I host a medical minute on Doug's television show, and you can watch me. I'm on usually every day or two. The channel in your area differs, but you can watch his program online right now, just go to his website, *www.knowthecause.com*

Chapter 7
Itchin' For A Cure- Avoiding Dry Skin

You already know that you need to keep your skin hydrated, and I have lots of suggestions to help you do just that.

In your quest to maintain hydration, I want you to do this mindfully okay? Don't slather on any old garbage lotion for the sake of temporary relief, because there will be backlash on your skin. Some products contain all sorts of poisons, and I'll leave it at that. For more on what's in your lotions, you can visit EWG's Skin Deep website which allows you to search the database and find out exactly what's in your toothpaste, shampoo, lotion, make up, and so forth. In particular, I want you to avoid synthetic perfumes (essential oils are okay and natural scents). Avoid anything containing parabens, phthalates, and harsh sulfates.

There are dozens of clean companies that make chemical-free lotions. I may not have eczema, but I can certainly speak to this dry skin thing because I live in a desert region of the United States, so I'm constantly trying to keep my skin soft and moisturized, especially in the winter.

I've easily spent a thousand dollars trying lotions of every sort, and while I'm not an expert on every single ingredient, I can tell you these are my absolute favorites of the bunch. (Oh, and feel free to email me with your own personal favorites, my email is info@suzycohen.com). These are in no particular order, just as they fall out of my brain or I pull them out of my bathroom cabinet!

Naturopathica Aloe Replenishment Gel. Naturopathica is one of my all-time favorite companies for skin care. Everything they make is pure, soothing, and healing.

Their Aloe Replenishment Gel is a strong anti-inflammatory that contains aloe vera and prickly pear cactus, both of which have moisture-binding attributes. Aloe helps with redness and inflammation (even when caused by UVB rays). It supports the skin's natural immune system and therefore helps with visible signs of aging.

Aloe also repairs natural collagen. which is damaged in people with eczema due to the destructive enzymes released during inflammation. (You know those destructive enzymes as cytokines or what we call "soldiers" in my book. Aloe contains hyaluronic acid, which helps plump the skin.

This is a great product for anyone who spends time in the sun, and especially people with skin sensitivities. Visit *www.naturopathica.com* for general information.

I should mention that having a good old fashioned aloe plant can be wonderful too, just clip off a piece, squeeze it onto a painful, itchy area, and it should be very soothing. These plants are worth their weight in gold. Buy one at any nursery or garden center.

Hugo Naturals All Over Lotion. The delicious scents alone will make you long for this product. I take it to the salon when I get a pedicure so they can use THIS lotion, instead of their perfumed stuff. Hugo's is a company dedicated to purity and quality. They blend olive and jojoba oils with shea butter to make a creamy lotion. Some of their lotions contain vitamin E and aloe vera. Try the Lemon Verbena & Bergamot, or the Sea Fennel & Passionflower scent. Here's the website: *www.HugoNaturals.com*

Sumbody Hydrate Lotion. I found this little boutique called Sumbody while strolling the streets of Sebastopol, California. They make really nice products, such as a pure skin and face care line that is just incredible.

I like their lotion which contains avocado, coconut. and sweet almond oil along with Japanese honeysuckle, vitamin E, and grape seed. It's scented with a blend of delicate essential oils. Here's the website: *www.sumbody.com*

Magoroku Skin Lotion by Dr. Ohhira's. I know I've already mentioned probiotics, but I really think they are the key to good skin health. This lotion is thicker than traditional lotions. It's a little oily upon initial application (from the equine-derived oil), so it is instantly soothing and relieving to sore, inflamed areas. The makers combine probiotics and pre-biotics along with wild fruit and vegetable extracts for a blend that is unmatched. If I had eczema, I would live on this lotion, and apply it all day long. It promotes radiant looking skin and I believe with all my heart that restoring lactic acid bacteria to your skin, will drive out pathogenic bacteria, right at the sight of action.

This lotion contains alpha linolenic acid and linoleic acids, which cannot be made in the body. It's ideal for very dry and sensitive skin, and safe for the face. I personally use this on my heels when they get dry.

You can learn more about it the company's website *www.EssentialFormulas.com.* It's sold at certain health food stores and online retailers but it's not that easy to find because it's a specialty product. I have another idea, you can buy this lotion at the following site, and use coupon code "suzy12". Then you'll receive free shipping, and a free bar of Kampuku beauty soap, which I recommend for people with eczema. More information about Kampuku is coming up too, but in the meantime, if you want the lotion, or probiotics, visit: http://bit.ly/LK4hiI

Nubian Heritage's Coconut & Papaya Lotion. It smells divine and offers superior, lasting hydration; it also contains vanilla bean extract. This company makes plain Raw Shea Butter lotion. By the way, shea butter originates from the karite nut tree, a.k.a. the mangifolia tree, so it's not an animal source. I found these products at iHerb and Amazon and also at Whole Foods.

Aveda's Botanical Kinetics Hydrating Lotion. It absorbs quickly and contains emollients derived from coconut, jojoba. and other naturally-derived ingredients. You can find it at salons and online. This particular lotion replenishes moisture gently, and I like that it contains chamomile and lavender essential oils. Here's the website: *www.Aveda.com*

Skin Talk: Immediate Treatments for Relief

Here are some general tips to help soothe swollen, red, itchy skin. In case you didn't realize it, your skin is the largest organ in your body! Your skin is the external manifestation of what is going on inside of you. If you look at a plant, you can usually tell what the plant needs--more water, more sunlight, less sunlight, etc. Your skin, as well as your hair and nails are likewise a good barometer for your internal health, so pay attention.

Bear in mind that itchy skin can be part of the eczema picture. When that itch is chronic and inexplicable (as opposed to poison-ivy induced), it means your immune system is unhappy with something you're exposed to, such as detergents, cosmetics, sunscreen, latex, nickel, medications, pet dander, or a particular food. We discuss immunity and allergic reactions elsewhere in this book. Here let me do what I do best, walk you down the aisle of my virtual pharmacy and show you what you can use to soothe your skin. I'm not sure what's right for you, so ask your doctor, or try a testing on a small patch of skin before applying liberally. (And remember, none of these are.)

Here's a look at what's in inside the most popular anti-itch remedies:

Hydrocortisone. Dozens of creams, ointments, sprays, and roll-on products contain this steroid, which helps control the itching, redness, and inflammation associated with skin rashes, eczema, psoriasis, bug bites, poison ivy, and seborrheic dermatitis. You can ask your doctor to call in a stronger prescription strength, or a sister-steroid like betamethasone, but these will have to come from your pharmacist (after your physician phones in the script). Lower doses of hydrocortisone are sold OTC at any pharmacy. You can apply every 3 or 4 hours as needed. Please refer to Appendix 1 for a more complete list of topical steroids.

Domeboro. This is powdered aluminum that you mix with water to make a compress, dressing, or soak. It acts as an astringent on the skin and comforts skin rashes, bug bites, athlete's foot, poison ivy/oak, or poison sumac.

For any kind of acute, weeping, or oozing rash related to eczema, a soothing wet Domeboro dressing or baths could help relieve the inflammation and itching. For acute and localized eczema, you can certainly use Domeboro powder, or Bluboro powder; just follow label directions. Domeboro is my choice of these two because the active ingredients are the same (aluminum sulfate, calcium acetate, boric acid) but the Blueboro powder also has FD&C blue coloring. (Please tell me why they have to take a perfectly good product and mess it up with synthetic additives, but anyway...)

Aveeno bath. Imagine soaking in oatmeal, except you can't add blueberries and cream. The packets of natural colloidal oatmeal are intended to be sprinkled into your bath water so you can soak your irritations away. It helps with itchy skin, rashes, eczema, insect bites, and poison ivy/oak or sumac. Many people on the Internet suggest using Aveeno bath oil, or another similar product called Alpha Keri Bath Oil. These would not be my recommendations because their primary ingredient is mineral oil, derived from petroleum, and I'm not loving that even though many experts do feel it is the least irritating oil to apply to skin. Nah, I think coconut oil is miles better and it has antifungal properties to boot.

Soothing oils. Apricot kernel oil may be particularly good for relieving itch in certain people. I like either coconut or apricot kernel much better than anything containing mineral oil. There are two other oils that I want you to look into. One is organic grape seed oil; the other is tamanu oil. These are made by various manufacturers, and if you have your own favorite brand go with it. The company I like is Aura Cacia, and they make both of these oils.

Tamanu oil comes from Tahiti, and it should be cold-pressed. All of these oils, whether you choose coconut, apricot, grape seed, or tamanu are remarkable topical healing agents because they support skin healing, and have an antineuralgic, anti-inflammatory, antimicrobial, anti-fungal effect on the skin. They are antioxidants too, sweeping away damaging free radicals. Now you can see why I prefer these oils to mineral oil, or petroleum based lotions.

Sarna Sensitive. This lotion contains pramoxine, which basically numbs irritations and relieves itching for minor skin irritations. Sarna's "original" version is very cooling because it contains menthol and camphor. It's not something to slather on all over, but it could instantly soothe small patches of skin that annoy you.

Calamine. I'm talking about the pink lotion traditionally used to relieve chicken pox and poison ivy lesions.

It's a skin protectant that dries oozing and weeping sores while relieving minor pain and itching. It's great for relieving the itch of eczema. The Calamine Plus version is stronger because it contains pramoxine along with the calamine.

Clay. YES! I love clay. Get either Bentonite, French Green Clay, or Rose Clay. There are whole books on this topic, and websites devoted to how these are derived and what action they have on the skin. Clay may be one of the most affordable, simplest, and effective treatments. I could not love clay anymore; in my house, I always have some on hand.

You can buy clay commercially prepared, or you can buy powdered clay and just make it at home with a little plain water, or rose water, or even coconut oil (or olive oil). The point is to make a paste of it, apply it to your skin and let it do what it does best, draw out toxins from your skin and soothe it.

Since I'm a mad scientist myself, if I were making the clay, I'd use the Bentonite, mix it with plain water, and add 2 drops of lavender essential oil. I'd leave it on my skin for an hour and then remove by rinsing gently under warm water (no soap). I'd do this a couple of times daily. Earlier, I mentioned putting some clay into your bath, about 1 cup per bath (and you can mix it with Epsom or Dead Sea salts if you want). Buy ready-made Bath Salts Plus by Redmond Trading. This product is sold online and you can ask your health food store to order it for you if you wish.

If you buy off their website, they give my fans and friends a discount. Go to checkout at their site and put in my name "suzycohen" it will give you 15% off your entire order. Just as an aside, if you spend more than $35 USD, you get free shipping (however, you have to take into account the 15% discount which may cause you to fall below the $35). *www.RedmondTrading.com*

You can try also try this simple home remedy which I highly recommend for acute flares. Take about 1 tablespoon of clay, and hydrate it with Silvercillin. (*Designs for Health* makes this and it's sold at holistic doctors' offices, some health food stores, compounding pharmacies, and online retailers.) You can certainly use any other brand of nanosilver, or colloidal silver that you like. For every tablespoon of clay, you'll need approximately a teaspoon or two of the silver solution because you want it on the more pasty side, not dripping wet. I can't tell how much liquid you need, but the point is you want to make a paste that you can apply about 1/4 inch thick. Cover it with a cotton dressing. Change it every day using fresh clay. I've heard that this could help heal a patch of scaly skin within several days. Woo hoo! Also, applying nanosilver, or colloidal silver directly to your skin should be okay too. You can try that and see if you get faster results. The clay would be good to use if the eczema is oozing, because clay will draw the toxins out.

Silver is a broad spectrum antimicrobial, which also kills mold, viruses, and other bacteria. It should not interfere with your good healthy bacteria. The brand I referred to above (Silvercillin) also comes a liquid you can take internally. It also comes as a gel and a topical spray. You're welcome to try any or all, and let me know the results.

Zinc Oxide. Zinc oxide paste i. You may have seen it on the noses of people at the pool. Most people use it for their baby's rash, or to prevent minor skin irritations such as burns, cuts, poison ivy, poison oak or poison sumac. Zinc oxide can be helpful to soothe inflamed, irritated skin, especially if there is weeping fluid present, but you don't want to put it on large areas. Some people say that it's hard to rub in completely because of the residue. I've heard that some people are allergic to zinc oxide, but I have to wonder if that's really more of a sensitivity to another other ingredient in the salve, such as dimethicone, parabens, lanolin, oils, petroleum jelly, wax, etc.

DMSO. Unfortunately, I cannot elaborate on this ingredient, because it is so controversial. Dimethyl sulfoxide or DMSO is only approved for use only in horses to relieve pain, not humans. You have to buy DMSO over the Internet (for your horse of course), as it's not sold in health food stores because it is classified as a solvent. If you do a quick search on the Internet, you'll find that DMSO is commonly applied to human skin in order to relieve joint pain, fasciitis, bursitis, and tendonitis. It has a relatively safe side effect profile and efficacy. Many people use it successfully for its anti-arthritic pain-relieving qualities which is why it's commonly used for race horses! Did I mention it's *not* approved for humans even though humans use it every day?

There is always some DMSO in my house because I have a horse, no I'm just kidding with you about the horse. I applied DMSO to my knee just 10 minutes ago because I went a little crazy in yoga yesterday, so it's helping me. Seriously, DMSO could very well be the best kept secret. It is applied topically to manage minor aches and pains associated with athletic strains, tendonitis, plantar fasciitis, and so on. It is a carrier and will drive into the tissues, whatever you apply first, so I buy the roll-on version that is 70% DMSO. For me, I put a few drops of magnesium oil to the area that I want to relax, say a muscle cramp, or the bottom of my heel where I have plantar fasciitis, and then I roll the DMSO on top of that. It drives into the tissues all the magnesium, plus it works in and of itself.

As for skin conditions, depending on which one, DMSO may be helpful. I can't tell you personally what to do with a non-FDA approved solvent for your eczema. That said, there is some research to suggest DMSO applications can help with mild eczema.

You do not want to apply too much of it to broken skin. Or perhaps you want to do a skin patch test, just apply to a small area (like a quarter inch area), and see how it feels. Just read up on your own, as this particular product is one worth mentioning, but you have to make your own decisions. I went to a website called www.dmso.org and found some intriguing stuff.

Random Skin Tip: Autoimmune Progesterone Dermatitis
Some women have eczema concerns cyclically. They experience flare-ups about a week before the beginning of the menstrual flow (it could actually be 3 to 10 day), and it magically clears about 2 days into menses. This is not true eczema. It's actually an autoimmune disease known as "Autoimmune Progesterone Dermatitis" or APD. I would suspect that this is a Th1 dominant condition, whereas true eczema is Th2. (I go into a great deal of detail about Th1 and Th2 conditions later in this book.)

Chapter 8
Could It Be Your Medicine?

You need to see your doctor to help you determine what is causing the prickles. Even if you take medicine for years, you can suddenly become allergic to it. Your doctor may suggest a "drug holiday," during which you wean off all medications and go without them for a few weeks, then begin taking one drug at a time to see whether a particular drug is causing your problem. Drug holidays should never be attempted without your doctor's agreement and supervision. Some medications are necessary to maintain heart rhythm, and others must be discontinued slowly, not abruptly.

Medications that could be fueling eczema flare ups, include the following:

Antibiotics

Antifungal drugs

Antiviral drugs

Anti-parasitic drugs

Antihistamines

Phenothiazines

Steroids

Non-steroidal anti-inflammatory drugs

Anesthetics

Chemotherapy

As an aside, it's good for you to know that drugs can rob your body of essential nutrients. I call this the drug-mugging effect and have written a book on this topic explaining which vitamins and minerals you should be taking, if you are on a particular medicine. Paying attention to this issue can save you from getting diagnosed with a new "disease" when you are just experiencing a side effect because of the drug-nutrient depletion effect. For more information about my Drug Mugger book, you can go to Amazon and read reviews.

Because biotin, B6, and folate are 3 important B vitamins that protect your skin, it's worth noting that various medications seriously mug you of these. Also, silica, iodine, zinc, vitamin C, selenium, magnesium, and calcium all play a role in hair and skin integrity. Guess which classes of medications are able to reduce levels of those important micronutrients? All of the following are world-class drug muggers of skin-loving nutrients. So if you're on any of these, ask your doctor if you can switch medicines (to a totally different therapeutic class), or at the very least, take vitamins to put back what medication stole. Here's the short list; the lengthy one is my Drug Muggers book:

Acid blockers- Used to decrease acidity in the stomach

* H2 antagonists (ranitidine, famotidine, cimetidine)

* Proton Pump Inhibitors (omeprazole, esomeprazole, lansoprazole, rabeprazole)

Antibiotics- All of them; there are hundreds!

Oral contraceptives- Used to prevent pregnancy and stabilize erratic cycles

* The Pill (all brands, even the mini-pill)

* The patch (Ortho Evra for example)

* The shots (Depo Provera)

Hormone Replacement Therapy or "HRT"- Used for menopausal symptoms

* Creams (Premarin cream or Estrace)

* Pills (FemHRT, Estradiol, Prempro, Premarin tabs)

* Vaginal ring insert (Estring)

Corticosteroids- For allergies, asthma, autoimmune disorders & chronic pain

* Prednisone, prednisolone, methylprednisone, hydrocortisone

Alcoholic beverages

Coffee

Refined sugar or processed foods

Chapter 9
Eczema Be Gone! What Else Can You Try?

So far I've given you long list of things you can try and foods to avoid.

I'm not done giving you options! Here are a few more helpful hints:

Coal tar products. Coal tar is a black sticky liquid produced during coal distillation, where they heat the coal in the absence of any air. They are anti-inflammatory or antimicrobial in nature. This byproduct also serves as a natural moisturizer and is sanctioned by the American Academy of Dermatology to effectively reduce redness and sooth itchy skin. You can buy coal tar soap and skin care products everywhere.

Be aware that coal tar has a little odor. You will want to rinse it very thoroughly. Coal tar remains active for about three days after application; however, follow label directions for your product. It is not without limitation. You should never apply coal tar soap to infected areas, blistered skin, or anywhere where blood or pus is present. This stuff will stain your clothes (and skin temporarily) so please be careful applying. It makes you a little more photosensitive so you may need sunscreen if you spend a lot of time outdoors. (Don't get me started on the sunscreen rant here, I have to focus on eczema).

Read your labels carefully because there are products that are sold OTC that contain only coal tar fragrance, as opposed to actual coal tar. Tricky tricky! You have to read the label before purchasing a product to see if it has your desired ingredient. Also, be aware that if you have very sensitive skin, coal tar products can make problems worse, rather than alleviating them.

For many reasons, coal tar products are not among my favorites; however, I think they have some temporary value because some of my customers at the pharmacy used to rely on them. Knowing that eczema stems from a deeper problem inside of you, versus a skin problem, I don't consider them to be a long-term fix. Let me just say, for the long-haul, they are not my cup of tea. Speaking of tea...

Oxalates. You might want to try easing back on dietary oxalates and see if that helps. Oxalates are found in lots of different foods, including black and green tea, all forms of soy, all nuts and seeds, beets (even pickled), leeks, okra, spinach, sweet potatoes, Swiss chard, raw elderberry, gooseberries, amaranth, wheat, star fruit, and rhubarb. Other big offending foods that contain a lot of natural oxalate include chocolate, instant coffee, corn, beer, potatoes, and various beans. Obviously, this list contains a lot of foods that are otherwise considered healthy. What's the problem here?

Calcium oxalate crystals lodge in soft tissues and some experts suggest this drives skin problems such as eczema, as well as multiple food sensitivities and intolerances, diarrhea, migraines, and kidney stones. But there's always debate of course so let me head that off right here, right now.

When dietary oxalates bind to calcium in the gut, they handcuff the calcium available there, preventing it from zipping up the junctions between the cells on your intestinal wall. This is not a good thing because when those junctions aren't zipped up tightly, there are holes, and stuff leaks out that shouldn't! What stuff? Large proteins can leak through into your circulation, causing food allergies to dozens, if not hundreds of foods, spices, fruits, and vegetables. This is what people term "Leaky Gut."

This is why eczema is often seen in people who have poor intestinal flora, because the underlying assumption here is that a leaky gut won't process oxalates properly.

In fact, dietary oxalates are not your only source of oxalates. Other sources of oxalates include vitamin deficiencies, which lead to extra production of oxalates. Another possibility is genetic profile that causes you to produce more oxalates.(see below). Exposure to chemicals and environmental pollutants is also problematic.

In summary, when the calcium oxalate crystals escape the gut, you often see eczema. Well, that's one theory anyway. Healing the gut lining is important and there are whole books just on that topic. It's also important to promote healthy gut flora by taking good probiotics (oh boy, there I go again with the gut bugs). Increasing calcium and vitamin D supplementation may also help.

I do have a great all-in-one herbal solution for you. Natural marshmallow root tea (known botanically as *Althea officinalis*) may help soothe and promote intestinal inflammation that is frequently found along with eczema, and it serves to moisturize you from the inside out. This natural herbal mixture of marshmallow may quite possibly be the tastiest solution in my whole book. I made a youtube video to show you how easily you can make this yourself. I suggest about one-half to one cup of it once or twice daily, in between medications, but without regard to meals.

If the link does not work, go directly to *youtube.com* and put this title in the search box: "Health Benefits of Marshmallow Root Herbal Tea." Or put my name in the search box too. In 5 minutes, you'll know exactly how to make this soothing, nourishing tea.

Chapter 10
Problem Genes?

Some people just have a genetic predisposition to eczema, because they have a mutation in their DNA that makes them more susceptible to skin problems, as well as allergies and inflammation.

One of those genes affects how much of a substance known as MMP-9 (matrix metalloproteinase 9) is secreted. If there's a mutation in your genetic sequence, then certain of your immune system's cells (neutrophils and eosinophils) will make a lot of MMP-9, and then you are more susceptible to eczema as well as wheezing and asthma. I think most people with the MMP-9 mutation have asthma as opposed to eczema, but it could be either or both conditions. Thank your parents for that! And if you smoke, you affect this gene in a worse way, which really cranks up your likelihood to have lifelong eczema flares.

Another important genetic mutation for eczema sufferers involves a gene called filaggrin. This is a totally different mutation from the MMP-9 above. The short story goes like this: Mutations in the filaggrin gene greatly reduce the amount of filaggrin protein in your skin or lead to its complete absence.

Filaggrin is a protein that keeps your skin intact, so less of it results in cracks in the skin barrier. When that happens you are more sensitive to things, because the less filaggrin you have, the more exposure the lower layers of your skin will have to allergens, which are supposed to be kept out, thus causing eczema. It's kind of like having leaky skin!

Once the foreign material, meaning the allergen, passes through your defective skin barrier, it gets spotted by cells of the immune system in your body. And your immune cells do what they're supposed to do, they go on the attack. Their well-intended army assault to rid you of the bad antigen leads to inflammation of your skin and other allergic responses, including asthma.

There is a strong connection between eczema and asthma. If you, or your child is exposed to allergens via the skin, that exposure primes the pump, meaning it heightens the immune system reaction to go after that allergen more aggressively. This helps explains the coincidence of asthma and eczema seen in people all around the world.

Now, having this gene is not a slam dunk for having the condition, but it usually goes hand in hand with more frequent flare-ups compared to people who do not have the filaggrin mutation. If there's a mutation in your filaggrin gene, you are going to have that leaky skin problem. You feel the itch, the flake, the burn, the redness, and so forth. It's estimated that at least 50% of children with eczema and atopic dermatitis carry this gene.

If you want be tested yourself for this FLA gene, ask your physician to order a special lab test. You can consider the following labs. Send me feedback because I'm not familiar with them personally, as I am with many other labs:

Advanced Diagnostic Testing (ADx). Ask for the Filaggrin Genetic Test. The test requires a buccal (cheek) swab and some blood, and it takes about 9 days to turn around the report to your physician. Find more information at www.nationaljewish.org

Geisinger Medical Laboratories. The name of the test is the Progenotyper Filaggrin Mutation Detection Panel. requires a blood sample. The turnaround time is not specified at their website: *www.geisingermedicallabs.com*

I asked Jill C. Carnahan, M.D., the founder of *Flatiron Functional Medicine* in Boulder, Colorado, about these tests. She's a bit of sleuth in terms of detecting what is wrong with her patients. She said that she uses the filaggrin test for her eczema patients because it's good to know your genes.

"As long as you're testing yourself, why not opt for the Complete Atopic Dermatitis Panel, which includes common food IgE sensitivities, as well as yeast and bacterial IgE responses," urges . "People who have developed a chronic dermatitis on their scalp or suffer with persistent stubborn eczema will have IgG antibodies present in their blood, long after the bacteria or yeast have cleared from the lesions on the skin. The presence of these detectable antibodies perpetuates the inflammatory responses and slows healing."

I want to echo what she is suggesting here. In fact, one germ called *Staph aureas* is found in more than 90 percent of skin lesions. People with atopic dermatitis make specific IgE antibodies to the toxins produced by these germs and also fungal antibodies to Candida and Malassezi, two fungal species. Having antibodies to these organisms makes for a vicious inflammatory response if you are not vigilant about keeping these bugs at bay.

Itching Begins in the Brain Sometime!

Lucky you, if you happen to be one of those people with a low threshold that perceives itching faster than others. It's been shown in a 2008 study published in the *Journal of Investigative Dermatology* that itching is modulated in the brain. The authors concluded that the perception of itch really is regulated in your head. Some people are scratchy all over, while others won't notice it at all. A brand new study published recently in June 2012 issue of *Chemical Immunology and Allergy* reviewed current studies and concluded the same thing. Itch is in the brain, and if you have eczema, as well as a low threshold for itchiness, you're going to feel the maddening sensations more furiously.

Chapter 11
Nitty Gritty Stuff: Th1 vs. Th2 Immunity

Oh boy, I dislike getting all technical on you but this is truly the best time to tell you that high levels of a compound in your body called Interleukin 18 (IL-18) can increase the misery for you. One totally affordable way to reduce levels of IL-18 is with aerobic exercise. This was shown in a 2006 study published in *Brain Behavior and Immunology*. I love saving you money, and helping you feel better! So get out there and shake your booty if you like Zumba, jog around a local park, or get on your treadmill while watching "America's Got Talent." I don't care how you do it, just get up and sweat.

Now, here's the shocker heard round the world: Psoriasis and eczema must be treated completely differently. They are actually the opposites of each other! Does that blow your mind? Most people think those two conditions are similar, and that treatments are similar. It is confusing. As I was researching this book I saw the two disorders mentioned in tandem constantly. Over and over, I kept coming across sites that erroneously advocate using the very same supplements for both conditions. WRONG!

I'll explain this shortly, but in a nutshell, psoriasis is an autoimmune condition and eczema is NOT autoimmune. Psoriasis is a Th1 dominant condition, and eczema is a Th2 dominant condition.

Th1 stands for T helper 1.

Th2 stands for T helper 2.

Science is so complex at times. To put it simply, there are all kinds of "armies" in your immune system.

Your immune system, which resides in your gut for the most part, is made up of two primary armies composed of cells that go on the attack to defend you: The Th1 and Th2 armies. Picture those as a see-saw with Th1 on the left, and Th2 on the right. In order for your body to be healthy, you want the see-saw to stay level.

When Th2 is overactive, for example, it tilts the see-saw in that direction and contributes to allergies. In case you are having trouble visualizing that, let me say it this way: When Th2 is high, it automatically means that Th1 is low. Guess what? Underactive Th1 immunity contributes to yeast overgrowth.

The dietary supplements you take have an impact on driving Th1 or Th2. In other words, the supplements stimulate either Th1 or Th2. So the type of condition you have, should determine the type of supplement you should be taking. Most people pay no attention to this, and mistakenly take highly-touted dietary supplements that actually make them sicker.

Right here, right now, you will learn the general rule of Th1 versus Th2 dominance, and you will be able to outsmart everyone in your house, and possibly even your doctor, if he or she is unfamiliar with this aspect of immune function. Here's the rule: **Modulate Th1 and Th2 immunity so that there is BALANCE and neither is over-stimulated.**

Makes sense right? You don't want the see-saw to tilt too much in either direction because that means illness. Pretty soon, you will fully understand why certain dietary supplements are harmful and others helpful and why your best friend can take a supplement that you can't. It has to do with YOU, not the supplement, meaning it has more to do with whether a person has a Th1 dominant condition, or a Th2 condition, not how great a supplement is. Trust me, there are great supplements out there that are fabulous for some people and not so good for others. Take resveratrol, for example. This is fabulous for someone who is Th1 dominant, but not so good for Th2 people.

Emerging research indicates that inflammation is basic to the autoimmune disease process. During inflammation, your body releases a wide variety of chemicals (cytokines, eicosanoids, ROS [reactive oxygen species]), and other compounds that overwhelm your body. In other words, that see-saw in your body gets tilted. Stick with me here; we are just getting to the fun part. I need to remind you right now:

Psoriasis is an autoimmune condition.
Eczema is not autoimmune.

The take-away point here is that psoriasis is a Th1 dominant condition and eczema is a Th2 dominant condition. They are treated differently, just remember that. They are treated in opposite ways in fact. Which is why I got so incensed while doing research for this book! Some so-called experts are advocating that you treat your eczema with the very same drugs and supplements used for psoriasis. I'm just sitting here scratching my head thinking, NO!

As I sit here and type, I can just hear physicians telling me that in clinical practice this distinction is not so simple. For example, some patients have both eczema and psoriasis on different parts of their body. And the more data that comes out about Th1 and Th2 activation, they are led to believe that it may not be as black and white as we think. Yes, I agree; there are always exceptions in medicine. However, for all practical purposes, I'm keeping this book simple. If you have eczema, let's assume for today that it is not autoimmune (because for most people, it just isn't). There, I'm glad I got that off my chest.

Now, I swear, I'm keeping this simple, but I need to tell you one more important fact. A Th1 dominant response means that your T cells are attacking the antigen—that is whatever substance is triggering an immune system response. And a Th2 immune system response means that your B cells are mounting the attack and forming antibodies for you. Whichever it is, it's fair to say that this is a dynamic process. A blood test can determine whether you are Th1 or Th2 dominant. It's even possible that you can switch back and forth from time to time, during the course of your illness. You need to know if you are Th1 (T cell driven) or Th2 dominant (B cell driven) before taking supplements. And you need to know which supplements drive which part of the immune system. I'll teach you all that momentarily.

Psoriasis is almost always a Th1 dominant condition. In science speak, this means that cytokines such as IL-12 (interleukin 12), Tumor Necrosis Factor alpha (TNF alpha), and IFN (Interferon alpha and gamma), all stimulate the inflammatory response and create the fire in your skin. As part of treatment, you want to block those chemicals from forming. That's why physicians prescribe TNF blocking drugs such as Enbrel, Humira and Remicade. These drugs help by reducing one of the chemical soldiers (the cytokines) released in psoriasis.

Eczema, on the other hand, is almost always a Th2 dominant condition, so everything above does NOT hold. With eczema, the soldiers that work for the Th2 cells are known as Interleukin 4 or IL-4, IL-6, and IL-10. So you want to block those chemicals instead. I'm teaching you all this in case you want to go on the Internet and search "reduce IL-4 naturally" or "block IL-10, supplements," and you'll see what does that. I will give you the rundown of how to quiet Th1 and Th2 later. When you do that, you also capture those crazy soldiers and calm the flare-up.

Understanding Th1 to Th2 balance is important to you getting well. Unfortunately, this complex topic may never come up in your doctor's office, so I need YOU to understand it so you can take better care of yourself, and ultimately have the healing you dream of. Without this new knowledge of immune system dysregulation, you could make your condition worse by taking a fabulous supplement (or drug) that is not right for you because you are revving up the wrong army in your immune system. So listen closely.

Health food stores make millions of dollars selling immune-boosting supplements, such as medicinal mushrooms and green tea. These generally boost Th1 cells, and this causes your body to attack ITSELF with even more fury if you happen to have an autoimmune disorder.

They are being touted to help immune disorders and for good reason... and these are fabulous supplement. but and it's a big BUT... **if you are Th1 dominant (and you probably are if you have an auto-immune disorder such as psoriasis) then Th1 driving supplements might make you feel miserable or trigger a flare.**

Likewise, if you are Th2 dominant, as most people with eczema are, then certain supplements will make you worse because those drive up Th2 immunity (and you're already high). I'm in your head now, so I know what you're thinking. What are you going to do? Which supplements help eczema? Which supplements should you avoid?

I've provided a list below that outlines which conditions are Th1 dominant, and which are Th2 dominant. I need you to realize that you could shift back and forth between these states of immunity; it is dynamic, not stagnant. The see-saw is always moving. And don't freak out but I have to tell you the list below is not complete, and some diseases are a mix of Th1 and Th2 activation.

Like I said earlier in this section, some people have both eczema and psoriasis at the same time. They have both sides of the see-saw swinging back and forth on any given day. Please ask your doctor what he/she thinks, and also be mindful of your body. If you start a supplement that causes a setback, perhaps you fall into the opposite category. So discontinue any supplement that seems to be exacerbating the problem. My information below is intended to help you, to get you thinking, and hopefully to get you well, but it's not gospel. The body is an amazing thing, and we are all individual. You may not fall into the category that I've outlined here so use all information with discretion and good sense.

Conditions Thought to Be Th1 Dominant

Multiple sclerosis

*Rheumatoid arthritis

Uveitis

Crohn's disease

Celiac disease

Hashimoto's disease

Sjögren's syndrome

Psoriasis

Pancreatitis

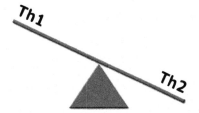

Type 1 Diabetes (may have a little Th2 involvement too)

Sarcoidosis

Chronic Lyme disease

H. pylori infection (this organism triggers ulcers)

Entamoeba histolytica

*Rheumatoid arthritis (RA) is generally thought to be autoimmune, but there are some cases that are related to Bartonella, a co-infection of Lyme disease. If you have RA, you should take a moment later on and read my article at my website, it is entitled, "Maybe You Don't Really Have Rheumatoid Arthritis" and you can find it by using the search box.

Conditions Thought to Be Th2 Dominant

Allergies & chronic sinusitis

Atopic eczema

Allergic dermatitis

Asthma

Nasal polyps

SLE (Lupus)

Mercury-induced autoimmunity

Scleroderma

Vaccination-induced disorders

Autism (but not always)

High insulin

Chronic fatigue syndrome or CFIDS

Fibromyalgia

Gulf War Syndrome

Malaria

Melanoma

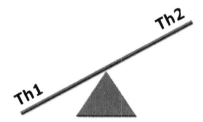

Helminth or other parasite/worm infection

Chronic hepatitis C

Chronic giardiasis

Chronic candidiasis

Cancer or dysplasia (cancer is a Th1 deficient state, therefore it is Th2 dominant)

Viral infections (HIV, HHV6, EBV, CMV, shingles etc.)

Ulcerative colitis or Inflammatory Bowel Disease

Food allergies (IgE mediated)

Pregnancy

Bringing Balance to the Th1 vs. Th2 Immune System

I'm so happy for you, because now you're easily on your way to healing your eczema by *just knowing that you're more likely to be Th2 dominant.* Now you have a better sense about which supplements to avoid, and which might help you. Trying new supplements will confirm this for you, because you will either start to get better, or you'll react badly and then you know. It's trial and error. I can't make any promises, nor can I advise you to do something. You must get your doctor's approval for all of this.

The only way I know to bring true balance to a tilted immune system is to nurture the GI tract, because 70 to 80 % of your immune system cells are in your gut. Seriously! You are sort of what you eat, or at least you will become what you eat! So nurturing that part of your body will make your skin beautiful. Let's talk about what your solutions are next.

Heal dysbiosis in your gut. Dysbiosis just means bad bugs in your gut. "Dys" means "abnormal" or "bad," and "bios" refers to the "life" or bug population in your gut. You can restore balance by driving out the abnormal ones with good ones. In other words, there are bad bacteria, fungi, or parasites living inside you that you need to reduce. You can do that with herbs (berberine, artemesia, mastic gum) or antibiotics. Honestly, there are whole books on this stuff. Keep in mind that berberine is also a strong natural supplement to reduce blood sugar so if you take it as a stand-alone supplement, monitor glucose levels.

Restore healthy bacteria and yeast. You do this by using probiotics and beneficial yeast (*Saccharomyces boullardii*, etc).

Eliminate leaky gut. This takes time, but you need to alter your diet and take supplements that rebuild the the lining of your gut. Some popular supplements for that include glutamine, N-acetyl glucosamine, Vitamins A and E, marshmallow root, IgG 2000 (a Xymogen supplement available from your doctor) or Gamma-oryzanol, which is a metabolite of ferulic acid, something that helps with cholesterol and gut lining all at once.

When you patch up a leaky gut, then big globules of food particles can't get through your gut and get into your bloodstream, where they create circulating immune complexes (CICs). CICs cause problems in far-reaching places, like the skin. Healing the leaky gut and all that goes with it could take months to years. Many good websites and books are devoted to this topic. Hopefully my pointers will get you started on the right track.

How Supplements Impact Th1 vs. Th2 Immunity

Below is a list that I've compiled to make it simple for you while talking with your health care provider, and also while shopping. I've created this list, separating the herbs and nutrients known to activate either side of the see-saw, either Th1 or Th2. This is what you should refer to when shopping and researching nutrients. Remember, it's not a hard fast rule.

Compounds that Stimulate Th1

Don't hold me to this, but make note that these are generally better for people with eczema while bad for those with psoriasis. Ask your doctor about them before taking.

Astragalus

Aged garlic

Beta glucan

Chlorella

Echinacea

Folic acid or the more active versions, Folinic acid or 5-MTHF (Look online or at Thorne Research or Xymogen)

Ginkgo biloba

Goldenseal

IP-6

Korean Ginseng

Lemon balm (*Melissa officinalis*)

Licorice root (glycyrrhiza)

Maitake mushroom

Neem

*Reishi mushroom (*Ganoderma Lucidum*)

Sea vegetables

Transfer factor

Vitamin C

Vitamin E

Compounds that Stimulate Th2 dominance

These are generally better for people psoriasis and bad for those with eczema.

Caffeine

EGCG (green tea)

Grape seed extract

Lycopene

Oils such as safflower, soy, canola, corn and sunflower could be a problem.

Pine bark extract

Pycnogenol

Resveratrol

White willow bark

Compounds That Modulate the Immune System

Think of all these supplements as part of the big picture. I think these are important whether you are Th1 or Th2 dominant because they are basic. They are both anti-inflammatory and immunomodulatory. They modulate the immune system.

That's why they are called "immunomodulatory" and that's different than immunostimulatory which "stimulate" or enhance the immune system activity.

Probiotics

Vitamin D

Vitamin A

Vitamin E

Colostrum

Boswellia

Pancreatic enzymes
Turmeric (or it's extract "Curcumin")
Essential Fatty Acids

Putting Things in Perspective

Since we're on the topic of inflammatory chemicals, it's important to know that the standard of treatment for psoriasis (and Crohn's and rheumatoid arthritis) is to prescribe TNF blocker drugs. The TNF stands for "tumor necrosis factor." You may know the medications as Humira, Remicade, and Enbrel. While these drugs are better for psoriasis, I have heard many patients with eczema tell me they were taking them and not doing better. This goes back to what I said earlier, psoriasis and eczema should (for the most part) be treated the complete opposite way You see, these drugs tilt the see-saw towards Th2. They are TNF blockers; that means they help people with Th1 dominant conditions like psoriasis. That's fine if you have psoriasis. But recall that eczema is probably a Th2 dominant condition. So these drugs won't do much for you if you have eczema, and in fact may actually trigger a flare!

So if you have eczema, and you're own this type of medication and not doing well, it's best to have a conversation with your physician about getting off properly, and trying something else.

For the same reason, the use of IV or oral corticosteroid drugs which calm an overactive immune system (prednisone or methylprednisolone) will not help a person with eczema long term, but could help someone with psoriasis. I'm just sharing my opinion, as it applies to the general population suffering with eczema. You see many of organisms potentially infecting their broken skin, so I don't think it's a good idea to dampen their immune system with corticosteroids. That said, sometimes in order to "stop the madness" and give the immune system a kick in the pants, caring physicians will give their patients a steroid medication for short term use, say 2 days to a week. This helps calm the severe flare of eczema. Once the immune system has been dampened down, the doctor can proceed to more natural root-cause type treatments.

You can discuss the use of all of the aforementioned drugs with your doctor. There is also a drug called Cellcept (the generic is Mycophenolate mofetil). It's a powerful immune suppressant, and it's only to be used by the patient to whom its prescribed. Others should not be exposed to this oral medication. To prevent exposure, the tablets should not be either crushed or opened. It's a strong medication, and I rarely recommend it. But you should know it is available.

Eczema is thought to be a Th2 dominant condition. All this means is that the Th2 part of your immune system is over-reactive, as compared to the Th1 part. You want these to be in balance.

When the Th2 immune system is hyper active, it causes inflammation, so the goal for you would be to drive down the Th2 army, and ramp up the Th1 army.

Another way to say this is that your Th1 immunity is suppressed, therefore you want to activate it a little more. And you can do this with herbs and dietary supplements! Are you happily surprised? A few herbs that could be helpful in waking up your Th1 immunity (and therefore calming down the Th2 immunity) is by taking a several of the following. Please ask your doctor what's right for you:

Koren Ginseng

Silica (I like Cellfood's brand of liquid silica)

Neem

L-glutathione (Preferably liposomal brand like Readisorb or Seeking Health. You can also try Xymogen's new tablet formula Acetyl Glutathione. You'll need to have your doctor order any of those for you.)

Do you want to be taking all of the above? Heavens no! Maybe try one or two, or even three and introduce new supplements one per week (or longer) so you can limit the amount of variables in your system and track effects.

Skin Tip: NAC for Asthma and Eczema

IgE antibodies are involved in eczema as well as hay fever, asthma, anaphylactic shock, and any allergic condition. Interleukin 4 or IL-4 is a factor in the production of IgE antibodies. A study by Bengtsson et al. published in 2001 showed that supplementation with NAC (and glutathione) could reduce levels of IL-4 and enhance immune function in a way that is good for people with eczema.

NAC stands for N-acetylcysteine, and it's manufactured by many companies and sold at every health food store. It's also included in some professional formula lines, such as Thorne Research's product Cysteplus. The dosage varies from brand to brand; it's about 500 to 1,200 mg once or twice daily.

There are a few things to avoid that may increase the activity of your already-overactive Th2 immune system including:

Caffeine

Green tea

Grape seed extract

Resveratrol

Oils including safflower, soy, canola, corn, and sunflower.

Tobacco

Heavy metals

Excessive progesterone

Melatonin (studies are conflicting)

Your Skin Problem: Is it Auto-Immune or Not?

Psoriasis is an auto-immune disorder, but eczema is not. This is confusing because these skin problems both involve the same uncomfortable issues. Dr. David S. Klein runs the Pain Center of Orlando and is a regular radio show personality.

I called him on his program recently, and I point blank asked him how to end suffering for people with eczema. He suggested using topical MSM (methylsufonylmethane).

MSM is a dietary supplement that is most often taken by mouth for joint pain. While it's an effective anti-inflammatory for arthritis, taking it systemically like this won't help a person with eczema because it doesn't get to the skin lesion (there is no blood supply); the blood vessels choke themselves off. So you have to apply the MSM directly to the skin in a high enough concentration to get the job done. The only product I recommend that has a high enough potency was formulated by Dr. Klein himself, and it's called Kink-Ease MSM Salve, available at www.stagesoflife.net

Dr. Klein suggested a general protocol that should be safe for everyone. Of course, I always recommend you consult your own physician for anything I myself or physicians that I've interviewed suggest. It's just always good to ask what over-the-counter remedies are right for you. Now, here is Dr. Klein's best plan of action to treat people with stubborn eczema. It includes the use of two natural products, castor oil and MSM. Start with castor oil. Apply it to your skin rash directly. Just pour a few drops out and rub it in with your fingers or a cotton pad. Do this 3 or 4 times daily for about 4 days. Then stop. On the 5th day, begin applying topical MSM (Kink-Ease lotion). Rub it directly to your affected skin areas, and do so 4 times daily. It should start to clear within a few days to weeks. When I asked Dr. Klein about using curcumin for eczema, he had this to say: "While it is well-known to help with psoriasis, curcumin doesn't do a whole lot for people with eczema. It's certainly safe to take, and it's an excellent anti-inflammatory, but it's more helpful for psoriasis, as opposed to eczema."

Chapter 12
Dyshidrotic Eczema

Dyshidrotic eczema is different than atopic eczema, which is what we've been talking about so far. Dyshidrotic eczema, sometimes called "hand eczema" because most people with dyshidrotic eczema have it in the hands, about 80 percent. The term dyshidrotic eczema can refer to conditions that affect the hand or feet. It can appear on just the hands, just the feet or both hands and feet.

This is a form of hand eczema that is much more common in women than in men. It starts on the sides of the fingers and appears as small itchy bumps and then slowly develops into a rash. The condition can also the feet as well as the hands, or sometimes it's just on the feet. Secondary bacterial infection is usually a complication with dyshidrotic eczema. Those of you that have this know that the condition tends to worsen during the summer months.

What you may call "Dishpan hands" is actually a form of hand eczema which happens in response to the constant wetting and drying of your hands. This breaks down your skin's protective outer barrier after a while. If you are prone to dyshidrotic eczema or are recovering from an episode, you need to avoid getting your hands wet so frequently. Perfumes and preservatives in soaps and irritants in household cleansers can also make symptoms worse. One hallmark of this condition is the onset of clear, deep-seated, blisters on the hands that occurs within a few days. It shows up specifically on the sides of fingers, the palms of hands and/or the feet. It could be the sides of the toes or the soles of the feet. These blisters may cause a burning sensation or intense itching.

Later, it starts peeling, cracking, or crusting and you may also see scaling, thickening, and painful fissuring occur. Chronic sufferers often have their fingernails affected, as in ridging, discoloration, thickening, pitting or other abnormalities.

Episodes can vary in frequency from once per month to annually, or every few years. Stress is definitely a trigger although there are other causes and contributing factors. For example:

- Cold or flu (speaks to immune dysfunction)

- Allergies: Food sensitivity, hayfever, etc. (this also speaks to immune dysfunction)
- Fungal infection (Yep, immune problems that allow fungus overgrowth)
- Diet (What you eat has bearing on your immune system... starting to see a pattern?)

These first 4 risk factors speak to the whole concept of immunity. As you learned earlier in this book, your immune system has 2 armies, Th1 and Th2. When either side of the immune system is tilted, eczema flares.

Here's what else triggers dyshidrotic eczema:

- Metal salts in the diet (foods high in chromium, nickel or cobalt).
- Times of Worry or Anxiety
- Genetic predisposition - Dyshidrotic eczema tends to run in families.
- Certain work exposures (e.g., cobalt) and/or recreational exposures
- Exposure to contact allergens (e.g., nickel, balsams, lactones) before condition flares

- Costume jewelry (because it often contains nickel)
- Cement workers, or any worker that touches either cobalt, nickel, chromium
- Wearing socks and shoes so that your feet sweat a lot.
- People who frequently wash hands (florists, nurses, doctors, restaurant workers, etc)
- Detergents, solvents and irritants that you touch. Avoid contact as much as possible.

Dyshidrotic eczema causes itchy fluid-filled blisters (called vesicles) on the hands, fingers and soles of the feet. It's sometimes called keratolysis exfoliativa or vesicular eczema. Most people just call it "hand eczema" but that's not technically correct because you could have regular atopic eczema on the hand. Dermatologists diagnose this usually by looking at it, but on occasion they will do a biopsy or skin sample in order to rule out the possibility of fungal or bacterial infection. I don't know why scientists have to confuse people but there are other names of it too:

Affecting the hands: Cheiropompholyx
Affecting the feet: Pedopompholyx

You may need an over-the-counter or prescribed antihistamine (like Benadryl, Claritin, Allegra, etc) to control the maddening itch. Benadryl should be taken at bedtime because it causes severe drowsiness and dizziness. All antihistamines have the potential to cause drying side effects such as blurred vision, dry mouth and constipation. The heart of histamine-related food sensitivities can cause dyshidrotic eczema (and regular eczema).

Earlier in my book, I mentioned a supplement that contains Diamine Oxidase or DAO. This is a must for people with dyshidrotic eczema in my humble opinion. And a low-histamine diet would also be in order for at least a 4 week trial.

Calamine lotion may help as well as any of the other soothing creams/ointments listed in my book. M recommendations for treatment would be exactly the same as for regular atopic eczema.

Unfortunately, there is no quick and easy solution to hand eczema unless you find yourself in the list above and can fix things right away (ie eliminate exposure to solvents, or stop wearing nickel-containing jewelry). Clearing up an episode of the condition can take weeks to several months, and you'll need to continue babying your hands for as long as a year even though they are symptom free. This is a good reminder that once you get it under control, stay vigilant with your diet so as to not introduce sensitizing foods that trigger flares. In other words, if you are among the lucky to get well, show your body gratitude by eating well and staying healthy.

Chapter 13
Castor Oil is a Comfy Alternative to Pain Meds

Many people apply castor oil directly to their skin rash, so you might wonder why wouldn't castor oil packs applied to the liver and abdomen area benefit you too? That is the traditional way to apply a castor oil pack you know… to the liver. And so yes, you're right, it would be a wonderful soothing option for people with severe eczema, and it's a rather inexpensive treatment. We haven't spent any time on this topic in this book, but please know that you must support your liver health if you have eczema. Your liver is overloaded with toxins and the better you clear toxins, the healthier your skin will be. Think of it this way, if you are loaded with internal toxins, one of the ways they come out of you is through your skin, so your skin is a reflection of toxins inside. And your liver is the organ that breaks down toxins. I wrote about the proper use of castor oil packs in a syndicated column and was inundated with weeks with questions about how to make one properly.

Castor oil packs can be particularly beneficial for women on their monthly cycle because they help with cramps. **Castor** oil packs are a safe, natural alternative to relieve many aches and pains. Keep in mind the heat will increase blood flow and so it may be contraindicated for you, or it could make your period very heavy and make you bleed like crazy, so either apply it the week before your period, or right after. If you apply it during your period be careful, perhaps no longer than 10 minutes or it will increase your blood flow.

I frequently recommend castor oil packs because they're non-medicated, have no side effects, and the moist heat feels good instantly.

Castor oil is rich in oleic and linoleic acid; it contains a strong anti-fungal, anti-microbial compound. That's why it helps with certain skin problems (keratosis, ringworm).

Castor oil is a vegetable oil that comes from the castor bean, which is actually a seed from the plant, *Ricinus communis*. India leads the global pack for production. As far back as 4000 BC, castor seeds were found in Egyptian tombs; the famous medical clairvoyant Edgar Cayce recommended castor oil in many of his readings.

Naturopaths can't agree on this, but I feel that castor oil should only be applied to the skin, *not taken internally*. An ideal location to apply the pack is on the right side of the abdomen over the gallbladder and liver, because this promotes bile flow, which relieves pain from digestive disorders. If you suffer with chronic pancreatitis, a castor oil pack may feel good. Women who get Mittelschmerz (ovulation pain which is mid-cycle) enjoy the warmth of a castor oil pack just below the belly button.

You will need a bottle of castor oil and a piece of wool cloth, about 12 by 12 inches. These items are sold at health food stores and natural grocers. You'll need some clear plastic wrap, or a plastic bag. Squirt the castor oil onto the wool pad. Saturate the cloth, but don't make it dripping wet. Warm the castor oil-saturated cloth by microwaving it 30 seconds. Careful, it gets hot very quickly. Apply the pack wherever your pain is.

Cover the wet cloth with the plastic wrap, and then put a little dish towel over it. Then, put a hot water bottle on top to keep the pack warm while you lie back and rest. Leave it on for 30 minutes to an hour, and repeat applications several times a week. Never apply to open (bleeding) wounds. To remove the oiliness from your skin afterwards, use a mixture of water and baking soda.

Chapter 14
Iodine: One Amazing Mineral

I asked Dr. David Brownstein, one of the world's leading authorities about iodine. David and I hosted a worldwide event on thyroid disease in the summer of June 2014, called The Thyroid Summit. (www.thethyroidsummit.com) I asked him if iodine played any role with eczema. After all, he is also the author of Iodine: *Why You Need It, Why You Can't Live Without It.*

Dr. Brownstein wanted me to relay this to all of you: *"The skin holds about 20% of the body's store of iodine. I have found many skin disorders--eczema, psoriasis, and others-- improve with it. Eczema is significantly improved with iodine, especially after clearing out food allergies."*

Just so you know, iodine is mugged by bromide, brominated vegetable oil, chlorine, and caffeine-containing beverages.

You will want to restore your iodine stash if you are prone to skin conditions, and especially if you drink those popular sports electrolyte drinks (can you please just stop drinking this stuff now?!), or if you swim laps in pools containing chlorine, or take frequent baths with Dead Sea salts that contain bromine. It's okay to bathe in those, I use Dead Sea salts myself sometimes, instead of Epsom salts (magnesium sulfate), because I think they are wonderfully soothing for the skin. But not all the time. It's the magnesium and the sulfur in Epsom that you really want. So I'm telling you that if you bathe in Dead Sea salts nightly (as opposed to Epsom), or even three times a week, the bromine in salts is going to reduce your skin's iodine level. So you just want to supplement with iodine in order to maintain optimal skin health.

There are many high-quality iodine supplements available and keep in mind they are helpful for breast health too. Getting the right amount is important. In case you didn't realize, iodine is a drug mugger of niacin, so if you get too much iodine you can mitigate some of the side effects with niacin.

Just for your safety, avoid high doses of iodine until you've consulted your physician to make sure it's okay. Also, you want to take smaller doses or avoid iodine if you have Hashimoto's thyroiditis or Grave's Disease.

Just run everything by your doctor, because while I help you fix your skin, I want you to feel great in all the other ways too.

Many people test their iodine levels using a skin test where they apply iodine and watch how fast it disappears. Don't bother; these test kits are like a magic trick. They are pretty much positive on every single person, and many factors come into play anyway. Your physician can offer you a urine test for iodine if you really want to test, and this is more accurate.

Let's spend a moment on iodine because there's another connection to your skin beyond simple levels of iodine. That is, if you run out of this important mineral, you could develop hypothyroidism, and that will cause or contribute to all sorts of other skin problems.

Iodine is one of the components that helps make thyroid hormone. It starts out as thyroxine, or T4 for short. The "4" refers to the number of iodine molecules bound on to the "T," which stands for "tyrosine." Thyroid hormone is just iodine and tyrosine glued together.

At some point, one of the iodine molecules leave, and you're left with T3, which is your body's fuel. T3 wakes you up and burns fat; it makes you pretty. Doctors can't agree on what the best range is.

You should feel pretty well if your T3 is between 3.5 and 4.2. This is another topic that could occupy a book which I will write for you one day. The point is to help you understand that proper thyroid hormone levels lead to happy skin. So get your levels into this range, and I think you'll feel a difference.

If you are tired, and holding weight, please refer to my article on iodine and thyroid health at my website entitled "Thyroid Health 101" and you can find it at my website, *suzycohen.com*.

The thyroid gland is the only part of the body that has cells capable of absorbing iodine, which it gets from food, iodized salt, and seaweed, but it doesn't get nearly enough. I was shocked when I learned that the *American Thyroid Association* reported that approximately 40 percent of the world's population remains at risk for iodine deficiency.

I think part of the problem is that foods grown in mineral-deficient soils are less nutritious. Bring in chemicals called halides such as fluorine, chlorine and bromine and you have a bigger problem on your hands.

These chemicals can crash your thyroid gland. These halides are annoying bullies and race for the same spot on the cell that iodine does; the bullies win.

Who are the bullies? For example, a very popular sports electrolyte drink contains bromine, your pool and jacuzzi contain chlorine, and most toothpastes contain fluoride. The problem is not coming from any one punch; it's the cumulative effect. Put all these things together and your thyroid gets upset. These bully halides are drug muggers of your iodine, and they could cause deficiency. This increases your risk for becoming hypothyroid, and what does that mean?

Too little thyroid translates into hair loss, depression, always feeling cold, weight gain, brittle fingernails, constipation, and pale, dry skin. Did I mention fatigue? Oh yeah, it's constant, and you wake up only after that triple shot latte. Iodine deficiency is not always the only cause for hypothyroidism. Your doctor can test you. Don't take iodine indiscriminately, because it can cause hyperthyroidism and nodules. For more information on thyroid (and iodine) please read my other book, "Thyroid Healthy."

You can also find more information at www.TheThyroidSummit.com which is an online event with 3 free hours of interviews on thyroid, hormones and iodine.

Chapter 15
Antihistamines to the Rescue?

There is a solid connection between eczema and high histamines, so an antihistamine may very well become your best friend. But these drugs, Claritin (loratadine), Benadryl (diphenhydramine), Allegra (fexofenadine), Zyrtec (cetirizine), and so forth, are not to be relied upon forever. They are just quick fix-me-ups. The pharmacist in me applauds the makers for offering people immediate relief with their drugs. The other side of the coin is that drugs only mask the histamine production. They don't cure the underlying cause. And you just become dependent on the drugs for partial relief, when you should be digging down deeper to find the ultimate triggers--i.e. metal allergies, food sensitivities, leaky gut, nutrient deficiencies, and so forth.

If you have eczema, eating foods that contain histamine may trigger an outbreak of the rash. Remember you are probably already making too much histamine to begin with, so taking in more histamine from your food is not a good idea. I've written about this later on in my book, and will offer you an incredible relatively new supplement (that contains DAO) that helps you beat the effects of histamine-related food intolerance. We'll get to that later on, for now stick with me.

Just as a reminder, histamine is a hormone that you naturally produce. While it helps defend the body from potential infections, you make a boat load of this histamine when you come into contact with thing you're allergic to. Imagine sneezing uncontrollably when exposed to pollen, cats, dust mites, sulfa drugs, penicillin, and so on. You get the picture. This is the reaction I'm talking about. So while your body makes histamine to help you, too much histamine (and/or another substance called leukotriene) may inflame your skin, causing eczema flares.

Typically, what you see with excess histamine is the following:

* Eyes itch, burn, or become watery
* Nose gets itchy, or you sneeze and produce more mucus
* Skin itches; you develop rashes or hives, or red, swollen patches of skin
* Sinuses become congested and cause headaches

* You experience wheezing or bronchospasms (Albuterol inhaler to the rescue!)
* Stomach problems; you may experience cramps and/or diarrhea

Histamine is a vasodilator. That means it's going to open up your blood vessels and cause redness and swelling very quickly. Remember how I told you that you might be eating nickel and exposing yourself to allergenic foods? Well, I'm going to tell you now that you might be eating high histamine foods. The following foods are high in histamine; and you will notice many foods that are fermented on this list. Fermented foods are generally a no-no if you are prone to skin problems. Here's the list, which I found at this website: *www.michiganallergy.com*

Table 1: Histamine-Rich Foods (including fermented foods)

These foods contain some histamine, so please limit or avoid until you know if you react to them:

- Alcoholic beverages, especially beer and wine.
- Anchovies

- Avocados
- Cheeses, especially aged/fermented cheese (Parmesan, Bleu and Roquefort)
- Cider and home-made root beer
- Coffee or black tea
- Dried fruits, such as apricots, dates, prunes, figs, and raisins (You may be able to eat these fruits without having a reaction if the fruit is thoroughly washed).
- Eggplant
- Fermented foods, pickled or smoked meats, sauerkraut,
- Mackerel
- Mushrooms
- Processed meats (sausage, bratwurst, hot dogs, salami)
- Sardines
- Smoked fish (herring, sardines, etc.)
- Sour cream, sour milk, buttermilk, yogurt (especially if not fresh)
- Soured breads, such as pumpernickel; coffee cakes and other foods made with large amounts of yeast
- Soy sauce
- Spinach, tomatoes

- Sunflower seeds, or sunflower butter
- Red wine vinegar or balsamic vinegar
- Mayonnaise (if it contains vinegar)
- Salad dressing, ketchup, chili sauce, pickles, pickled beets, relish, olives (it's the vinegar!)
- Yogurt

Histamine-Producing Foods

These cause your body to produce more histamine:

- Alcohol
- Bananas
- Chocolate
- Eggs
- Fish
- Milk
- Papayas
- Pineapple- Even though you see pineapples as a histamine-releasing food, you sometimes see its extract bromelain sold as a dietary supplement that works as a natural antihistamine. Fine by me, I like bromelain for people with allergies; you'll just have to see if it's right for you, by seeing if you get a flare
- Shellfish

- Strawberries
- Tomatoes

Momentarily, I'm going to tell you about something that contains "Diamine Oxidase" or DAO, and it's a supplement that can help you if you are intolerant to some of the foods above. But first, let's talk about traditional antihistamines, because that's what 9 out of 10 doctors recommend. In my book, these will be ineffective for many of you, however, for completeness sake, let's talk about them.

Other than bromelain, hesperidin, rutin, vitamin C and quercetin are strong natural antihistamines too, so consider adding one of those dietary supplements to your daily protocol. I really like quercetin. In order for quercetin to be effective as an antihistamine, you will need to take high doses. I recommend 1,500 - 4,000 mg daily. That is quite a hefty dose, so you may want to purchase the powder instead of capsules or you'll be swallowing caps all day long!
Obviously, if you take high doses, I want you to get your physician's blessings. Quercetin it is safe and effective for most adults, so just ask your doctor if it's right for you, or start with lower dosages and see how you feel.

There are other reputable brands of powdered quercetin that you can buy all buy yourself. If you find that it irritates your esophagus (and it shouldn't, but just in case), then go back to capsules and take a lower dose.

Let's hear it for stinging nettles, an herb-derived natural antihistamine with a long history of use. It is often used for urinary tract inflammation, enlarged prostate and regular allergies (like to pollen or grasses). You can buy it as tea, as dried herb (to make your own tea), and as dietary supplements that contain nettle, also known as as "Urtica dioica", usually a leaf extract. This is sold at health food stores, there have been some allergies, as there are with every herbal product, but overall the safety and tolerability of nettles is pretty good. I don't have any reason to take nettles but I tried it as part of my 'research' for this book. I am sort of experimental in personality and like to try things that I write about. I found that within 24 hours, I had a drying sensation of mucus membranes, but very gentle, and I felt a little more energy. I liked it, and think it could help some of you. Each product uses a certain concentration and potency, so I will not offer a dosage here, follow the label direction because the dose depends on how much the maker has concentrated the herb. If you grow your own, careful touching fresh nettle leaves, remember the name here, it's called "stinging" nettles for a reason. The safety record for this herb is good, although it has a blood-thinning effect (careful if you combine with gingko, ginger or warfarin (Coumadin), Plavix, aspirin etc). There are many studies online available at *pubmed.com* regarding it's considerations in other allergic conditions. It's well-studied, and can be beneficial to people with eczema.

Zinc is another simple inexpensive supplement to try, and you can buy tasty orange lozenges at any health food store or pharmacy. The dose varies, from 10 - 50 mg per day. Don't take too much, or you'll offset your copper ratio (suppress it), leading to bigger problems.

I would be remiss if I did not suggest digestive enzymes. There are supplements galore sold over-the-counter, and they are just intended to help you digest your meals. Some people, especially those with a history of allergies, often need a little helping hand in the digestion area. Taking a good blend of enzymes can dramatically reduce inflammation and stress on your immune system. I'm saying it can reduce the number of flare-ups you have, if you take the right enzyme.

Many people with rosacea, eczema, and psoriasis have found relief by including digestive enzymes in their diet. If you want a plant-based enzyme you can try Enzymedia's product called Digest Gold, which is one of my favorites. If you want a porcine-derived brand, try Thorne Research's blend called Dipan 9. Then of course, there is one popular brand widely sold at health food stores called Wobenzym N by Garden of Life. It combines both plant and animal extracts to help you digest your food.

The ultimate goal of using digestive enzymes is to reduce inflammation in the body, and so the brand doesn't matter much to me. You need to go by trial and error. What matters is how it affects YOU, and you should be able to tell within a few days of trying them.

You can take them in-between meals for a stronger anti-inflammatory effect, or you can take them with your meals to help you digest the proteins, carbs, and fats more effectively.

When Antihistamines Are Not Enough

Countless folks unknowingly suffer from food sensitivity and intolerance because the symptoms for it fall under the radar. Basically, it consists of various digestive system problems such as cramps, abdominal pain or spasm, diarrhea, constipation, flatulence and headaches. But it can also commonly cause skin rash and eczema. The reason is the body has trouble thoroughly digesting food that you eat, and that occurs do to a lack of certain digestive enzymes. So job #1 here is to be on a healthy digestive enzyme, I've talked about those just a minute ago. These sorts of supplements are usually taken on a 'trial and error' basis. You should know if it helps your condition within a few weeks. You take the digestive enzymes with your meals to help break down the meals (my choice for you, if you have eczema), or you can take them on an empty stomach to reduce systemic inflammation.

As you just learned, some people suffer because they eat foods that contain a lot of histamine in them. This is not a true food intolerance, it's more of an allergy. These elevated histamine levels can make eating pizza, fish, wine, beer and processed foods miserable for you. There are supplements that help, although I'd prefer you didn't eat high-histamine foods. See Table 1 for a list of "Histamine-Rich Foods."

Here's the chemistry. Histamine is an amine (nitrogen) that comes from a chemical reaction (decarboxylation) of the amino acid called histidine. In your digestive tract, the enzyme known as "Diamine Oxidase" often shortened to DAO breaks down histamine, and that is good. You want that DAO broken down.

If it's not you have too much histamine action going on. Elevated histamine can mimic the discomforts you get and think are immune system-based food allergies.

By taking a supplement that reduces histamine (and replenishes your body's own enzyme DAO), you reduce the risk for eczema outbreaks.

Two products that degrade histamine and quickly come to mind are "Histame" (*www.Histame.com*) and "HistDAO" by Xymogen (which requires you to have a physician order it for you, they don't sell directly to public because Xymogen is a professional formula line.)

For optimal results, take 1 to 2 Histame capsules within 15 minutes of consuming histamine-rich foods/substances known to cause food intolerance. Since the main ingredients have been developed to be stomach acid-resistant, you can open the capsules and swallow the ingredients (if preferred to swallowing capsules).

I think it's a brilliant, relatively safe thing to try but of course, ask your doctor if it's right for you. Unlike antihistamines, which only block the action of histamine, products that contain DAO help break down the bad boy, rather than block it's actions in your body. It's okay to combine both, meaning an antihistamine along with a DAO-containing product.

What you don't want to do however, is block your intestinal DAO and some of you do this because you require medications, or you take various supplements. Refer to Table 2 for a list of "Substances that Block Intestinal DAO" and see if you take something on the list. If you do, it means that you are blocking your own body's natural ability to break down histamine, thus it could cause a flare.

Drugs and Substances that Block Intestinal DAO (you want this)

- N-Acetyl Cysteine or NAC (used for breathing problems and to increase glutathione)
- Cimetidine, Famotidine, Ranitidine (acid blocker medication)
- Isoniazid (prescribed antibiotic)
- Verapamil ("Calan SR" a drug used for blood pressure)
- Propafenone ("Rhythmol" a drug for cardiac arrhythmias)
- Alcohol (sorry folks, any kind of alcohol, even the supposedly healthy red wine)

Food intolerance versus food allergy

It is important to differentiate a genuine food intolerance from a food allergy. The estimate is that 25 percent of our population suffers from this type of adverse reaction due to foods rich in histamine.

Food intolerance is a digestive system response to the inability to digest particular ingredients in food that does not involve the immune system. It does not trigger the Th1 army or tilt that see saw of immunity. In contrast, a food allergy is an abnormal response to food triggered by the body's immune system which perceives a particular food as a foreign particle and sends the Th1 army out to destroy it.

Reactions to histamine found in foods are not food allergies, though the symptoms can look and feel the same. Furthermore, the severity of the food intolerance symptoms is dependent on the ingested amounts of histamine-rich food. As well, symptoms of histamine related food intolerance can be controlled effectively with DAO supplementation.

Chapter 16

My Review of Popular Skin Creams and Potions

In this next section, I will give you a brief rundown of some popular creams and oils that could help you, and I'll be as blunt as possible because you are depending on me. I don't have eczema, but I can give you a good evaluation of what's out there, based upon ingredients, texture, and reputation.

First, I'd like to offer a recipe that you can give to your physician. Ask him or her to call this into the local compounding pharmacy where they can make it for you. If they can't make it exactly, it's okay; get something close. This is one amazing recipe that I think helps people with psoriasis and eczema. It's very soothing to the skin and applied topically.

You can make it yourself by buying all the ingredients separately (sold on the Internet or sometimes at health food stores). Making it yourself allows you to mix it in different ratios (for example, add more chamomile). Or you can do as I suggest and have your physician call it in as a prescription cream to the local compounding pharmacy, where it will be prepared for you--at a price of course, as this is a specialty item.

It takes time to order all this stuff in for a pharmacy so it's probably going to take a week to get everything in stock. I do not have any idea as to the price, but here's a working formula for you (or a natural pharmacist at a compounding pharmacy). These creams are all sold on the Internet. If you make it yourself, and that's what I would suggest since it's going to be hard to find a pharmacist to make it for you, don't worry about the percentages I've listed.

Just use an equal amount of each item--for example, 2 ounces of each ingredient--and mix it all together.

Suzy's Skin-Soothing Cream

Chamomile cream or ointment 1%

10 drops lavender essential oil

MSM cream or ointment 5%

Oregon grape bark extract 10% cream

Vitamin D3 cream 2%

5 drops Clary sage essential oil

Optional: Calendula ointment

Directions: Mix all this together. Apply as needed to skin rash. If you react, it's probably to one of the inactive ingredients in there, not to this recipe. For example, you may have to buy a MSM cream that is free of parabens.

Here are some commercially prepared products that you can also try:

Calendula Gel by Boiron. Yes, love this. Calendula (*Calendula officinalis*) is an herb that has been used safely all over the world for centuries, specifically for wound healing. A few European studies have concluded that calendula helps soothe wounds and improve healing. It has antifungal, antiviral, and even anti-tumor properties! I think calendula would be fantastic for cradle cap and diaper rashes, or any rash for that matter. You can use it on minor burns, sunburn, bedsores, eczema, and poison ivy. One small study even showed that it can ease the pain of radiation-induced dermatitis. Calendula may improve acne too.

Health food stores and online retailers sell calendula in cream, lotions, ointments, or tinctures. You'll see various brands and companies selling it, a few of which include Boiron, Weleda, California Baby, and Hyland's. I have Boiron's in my medicine cabinet as part of my first aid kit.

Even if you don't have eczema, but you are creating a first-aid cabinet, I highly recommend you include calendula. Put it next to your hydrocortisone and tea tree oil. Calendula is so safe you can literally eat the eat the beautiful yellow flowers from which the cream is made, so long as you're not allergic to flowers in the daisy or marigold family. Calendula extract imparts a beautiful yellow color, so it's used as a natural coloring agent in cuisines around the world. And, God forbid, you have eczema on your bottom or near your more delicate parts, calendula is not only soothing but very gentle to use.

I recommend Weleda or Boiron Calendula ointment for patients with psoriasis, eczema, or fissures, and it can do fabulous things for you! Also I occasionally recommend Alta Health Products brand of Pau d'Arco with Calendula ointment for anyone with stubborn fungal skin issues in the delicate parts.

Dream Cream by LUSH. No, not in love with this one. Many people recommend this on the Internet, and I've received letters regarding how effective this is, so I'm including it. It features a wonderful aroma and a smooth, silky texture. It contains oat milk, rose water, cocoa butter, glycerine, chamomile oil, tea tree oil, lavender oil, and a few other nice ingredients. My issue is that it contains two different kinds of parabens, propylparaben and methylparaben. It also has "perfume" listed on the ingredient label, perhaps explaining that wonderful aroma. I just can't personally endorse it because of the parabens; they are disruptors of hormonal function and thyroid production.

I'm including Dream Cream here because many people claim they get relief from this moisturizer. If you try it, you can let me know about results. It's sold by LUSH, from their website directly, and also by many online retailers.

Champoori Eczema Cream. Yes, love this. This is an all-natural herbal salve that I like to recommend for people with psoriasis as well as eczema. It contains all sorts of ingredients that support skin integrity, and I feel that it will be very nourishing. I've just heard from several people who tried it, how dramatically they improved, so I'm giving you the thumbs up on this product. You can go to their website and view before and after pictures of people who use the product. It contains glycerrhiza, phellodendron, and ledebouriella extracts. You apply it thinly 2 or 3 times a day to your problem areas. Here's where to learn more: *www.champori.com*

Botanical BABY Eczema Cream. Yes, I love this product. This is an all-natural herbal cream that I really like to recommend because it contains wonderful soothers like aloe, lavender, jojoba, sweet almond oil, calendula, seabuckthorn, rosehip extract, and zinc oxide. This is sold online.

Elocon Cream. This is sold ONLY by prescription. I like it for temporary use only, not forever, but it can really turn things around quickly with a bad flare. It is recommended that you apply a thin layer of the Elocon cream or ointment or a few drops of the lotion to the affected skin area once a day. Massage it in until it disappears, then wash your hands carefully so you don't get any residue in your eyes. Do not cover the skin with any plastic bandages or diapers, or occlusive dressings. The reason is that this will cause more drug to be absorbed by the body, and you don't want to receive more than prescribed. Long term usage of this cream can disrupt your body's ability to make your own natural adrenal corticosteroid hormones.

Most people tolerate this cream just fine; however, you are likely to experience minor side effects, such as some redness, blistering, burning, itching, or peeling. How that compares to your actual skin lesion is subjective.

Side effects occur most frequently when a large amount of Elocon cream is used for a long period of time. Potential side effects that you may experience include blurred vision, halos around lights, an irregular heartbeat, insomnia, mood changes, weight gain, or fatigue. If you experience any side effects while using Elocon eczema, it is important to notify your doctor immediately. Elocon belongs to the FDA pregnancy category C, which means this medication may be harmful to an unborn baby.

Natralia Eczema and Psoriasis Cream. Love this product! This is a homeopathic cream that goes on wet but dries into a clay-like balm that seals in moisture and soothes and heals with lavender oil, licorice, evening primrose oil, avocado oil, and zinc. This is a really helpful remedy for acute flares!

Chapter 17
What If You're Addicted to Your Steroid?

I know, this sounds ridiculous but addiction to eczema relief products does happens, and it's not to painkillers like you'd suspect. You should know that some people use topical steroids for minor skin conditions, and then it gets worse and worse. A sort of dependency occurs, and some people are apparently not able to get off them, and it's from the overuse. True story. There are ways to tell if you have steroid-induced eczema or genuine eczema.

5 Ways to Tell If You Have "Steroid-induced" eczema

1) You have used topical steroid drugs regularly for more than 4 weeks.

2) When you stop using your steroid cream or ointment, your skin turns red, or burns, swells, or begins to ooze again.

3) Your symptoms of eczema are getting out of control or spreading.

4) Your physician or dermatologist gives you different types of corticosteroids, or higher and higher strengths, but nothing gets that eczema under control

5) You've taken many tests for allergies and irritants, yet there is no cause and nothing to link to your flares.

Topical steroid-induced eczema can be cured. You just stop using the topical steroid. But before you do so, I suggest you get a different treatment plan or even a different dermatologist, because getting off the drugs is as hard as dealing with the resultant flare. You see, once topical steroids are withdrawn, the backlash begins for a while, and it could be painful.

So if you choose to withdraw from your topical steroids I highly suggest seeking guidance from a trained medical professional who understands the condition and has a better treatment plan. This is not to be undertaken by yourself. There is a worldwide organization devoted to steroid-induced eczema, they call themselves ITSAN for "The International Topical Steroid Addiction Network." They have a facebook page and the information posted there will help people with topical steroid addiction. *See Appendix 1 for a list of topical steroids and their respective potencies.*

Natural Oils for Big Relief

Commercial creams can bring relief. But please don't overlook the healing potential of natural oils. Here are several that may prove helpful:

Moringa Oil. I love this natural oil. It comes from an Egyptian tree. It's obtained by pressing the seeds from the *Moringa oilefera* tree, a fast-growing species sometimes referred to as the "miracle tree." I think there's good reason for that because so many people claim relief with moringa oil. I think the oil, which contains vitamin A, C, and radiance-boosting fatty acids, will help people with eczema. Moringa is a potent anti-oxidant, so it scavenges wrinkle-causing toxins in your skin cells.

One brand I keep around my cosmetic counter is "Moringa Oil" from Moringa Source. They make an entire line of beauty products. The oil is also sold by itself. You may find moringa oil sold as "Behen oil." There is another brand called "Ziga Oil," but that particular brand is an MLM product (distributed by a multi-level company) and I don't know anything about them. I'm mentioning it because a couple of my fans with eczema mentioned this product on my facebook page.

Clary Sage (Salvia Sclarea). This is incredible for skin problems, especially eczema and would be in any kind of lotion or ointment that I bought or made. In other words, if you buy a lotion or ointment, you can add the essential oil drops to it, thereby customizing your lotion. Medicinally speaking, if you inhale aromatherapy with clary sage, it seems to help relax the nervous system and improve memory, as well as improve mood and hormones. But as for the skin, the list is endless. It's an antiseptic, and it is known to improve acne conditions. It regenerates skin cells and eases the pain of boils and burns, allowing them to heal. It has anti-inflammatory properties so great for cuts and wounds. Are you loving sage as much as me yet? It is known to soothe skin conditions like psoriasis and eczema. If you have oily hair, put about 10 drops in your shampoo because it controls the production of sebum. It helps with oily hair, dandruff and even seems to discourage hair growth!

Blue Chamomile Oil (*Matricaria recutita, Matricaria chamomilla*). Yes, love this oil, it's a little pricey though. Just let me make sure to tell you that it's *not for internal use.* You dilute it in your bath water, or you dilute it with a carrier oil or lotion and apply to the skin. You can ask your massage therapist to put a few drops on your skin too, and rub it in with his/her regular therapeutic massage oil. For that matter you can mix up your own and take it to your massage therapist. The purpose of adding blue chamomile oil is to get the active organic compound known as azulene, which bears a natural gorgeous blue color. Azulene is a potent anti-inflammatory, and has many skin healing properties.

The blue oil actually comes from German chamomile, which has sedative properties. Blue chamomile oil may help people with acne, broken capillaries, burns, cuts, dermatitis, eczema, headache, muscular pain, muscular spasms, rashes, and nervous stomach. You can hunt this one down yourself, but it won't be easy.

I found blue chamomile oil sold by a few online retailers, Mountain Rose, which produces super pure products, is one of the best suppliers. I bought some and put 3 drops into my regular facial toner just for the benefits of it!

Vitamin E Oil. No, I wouldn't bother. It's not that vitamin E isn't soothing. because it is. But it's really hard to get enough of it to do any good when you apply it topically. I haven't heard anyone with much success doing this. You could however, take it by mouth. If you do, take a mixed tocopherol blend that says "natural." You want to avoid oral supplements that say d,l-alpha tocopherol because those are synthetic.

If you do decide to apply E oil to your skin, you can buy a commercially prepared oil at any pharmacy or health food store. You can also squeeze a capsule of it onto your skin too, but again, I'm not sure how well this is going to work for you. Hey, I promised you an honest review, didn't I? If you find a cure, or even significant relief with this one, do let me know via email. Instead of vitamin E oil, I recommend grape seed, coconut, or tamanu oil. Also argan oil, let's talk about that right now.

Argan Oil. Worth a try. This natural oil combines healing nutrients of other different oils that I like, such as almond, grape, olive, and avocado oils. You can put it directly on the skin. You do not have to dilute it by putting it in a mixer oil. I think this would be very soothing to sore, irritated skin. It is rich in fatty acids, so it moisturizes better than olive oil and shea butter, while helping with the pH of your skin.

I've read that Argan oil can reduce the appearance of scars from dried up eczema flares. Argan oil has both oleic and linoleic acids that have excellent soothing properties. It's especially good for applying around the eyes or mouth, a great option because steroid creams can be especially harmful around these areas.

It's a one two punch because it helps with eczema rash while also minimizing the appearance of lines. It doesn't happen overnight, but it can help.

Since I don't have eczema, I'm sorry that I can't report how effective it is going to be, but I can tell you that I believe in Argan's power, and after researching it, I suggest you give it a try. I have two types of Argan in my house. One I use just for moisturizing my skin during the cold, dry winters of Colorado, and another I spray on my hair to make it shiny and frizz-less. It smells so good, like almonds or something similar.

You can certainly research this, and find many products all over the Internet. You can ask at your local salon. Once in a while I see Argan at the local health food store. If you have trouble, or you just want to use what I use, I'll share that with you.

For the oil that I use on my face, I like to just put 2 or 3 drops in my hand with my regular lotion and spread all over, and sometimes I just put a few drops on my forehead or neck. This is what I use: Jose Marin's Argan Oil. It's sold at Sephora's and all over the Internet. It's free of parabens, sulfates, dyes, petrochemicals, and other junk; it's just pure Argan oil.

For my hair, I use Moroccan Gold Glimmer Shine Spray and it's on Amazon. Spray it from 12 inches away, just one or two sprays, because a little goes a long way. If you spray too much, you'll be oily. They make a serum too, if you prefer that to a spray.

Chapter 18

Looking at Light Therapy (Phototherapy)

Phototherapy exposes an individual to UV light, so if your eczema flares are related to sunlight exposure, this treatment is definitely not for you. , however, for many peopleThe treatments may include either UVB rays or UVA, or a combination of both. The rays may be narrowband or broadband. There is also one treatment specifically good for psoriasis called PUVA. In this treatment doctors combine the prescription drug Psoralen with UVA rays (hence PUVA).

When you take Psoralen orally, bathe in it, or apply it to the skin, it makes you more sensitive to UVA rays. One thing to know about this PUVA treatment is that the medicine stays in your eyes for awhile and so you have to wear UVA blocking sunglasses for 2 days after treatment.

The downside to any phototherapy is that you have to travel to a clinic where the treatment is offered several times a week. Another downside is that UV exposure is a known risk factor for premature aging and skin cancer. The point of the treatment is to give you some UV light at a specific wavelength so that it dampens down the exaggerated immune response that causes inflammation.

Phototherapy can help a person to reduce the dosage of medication and prevent bacterial infection, common in both psoriasis and eczema. If you opt for phototherapy, make sure you do your homework ahead of time. What I recommend is that you get natural sunlight exposure (without sunscreen) to your skin for about 15 to 20 minutes per day and less if you are extremely fair-skinned or have a history of skin cancer. This should provide adequate vitamin D to support healthy bones and immune system and may also calm your eczema flares without exposing you to risk of sunburn.

Chapter 19
Acupuncture Can Help

Now, this may seem counter-intuitive because if your skin hurts why would you want needles going into it? But you should and the needles likely won't go into the irritating rash anyhow. I'm a huge believer in acupuncture, and Chinese herbs. Try it, many people claim success. I won't claim to know exactly what to do, but if you find a good acupuncturist in your area, one that has experience with skin conditions, I think this can be helpful. I'm not of the mindset that needles have to hurt you while going in, in order for the acupuncture to be successful. It shouldn't hurt. If it does, I'd find another acupuncturist. I know I'm going to get it for saying that by some acupuncturist physicians for saying that, but that is how I feel (sorry). I've had about 100 treatments by 6 different doctors over the years, and the ones who hurt me were the ones I got the least benefit from, and obviously the most pain. I recall being told, "It has to hurt in order to get your Chi." Mild, minute pain is one thing, obviously there are needles involved, but a genuine hurt, or any kind of wiggling of the needle once it's inside... No! I disagree with there needing to be pain, and because I feel that acupuncture is incredibly valuable, if it hurts you or is uncomfortable, find another doctor. Don't give up. It can be enjoyable and enormously helpful in balancing out the Th1 and Th2 arms of your immune system.

Because I believe so much in the benefits of acupuncture, please remember, if you don't have a good experience the first time, or with a particular doctor, please try again, because the treatment and the care that you receive, differs with each physician. Actually, there should not be *any* real pain associated with this treatment. On the contrary, you should leave feeling more relaxed and better.

One study published in the *Journal of Alternative and Complimentary Medicine* found a beneficial effect from acupuncture combined with Chinese herbs. Twenty patients with mild to severe eczema were treated with acupuncture and Chinese herbs and then followed for 12 weeks. An improvement in eczema severity was noted in 100% of patients when compared to their baseline. On average the patients improved by approximately 64%. Not too shabby.

Deena, one of my fans from my Facebook community had this to say regarding acupuncture:

I went to an excellent acupuncturist who stuck needles all over my body for 3 days and gave me herbs. (Don't ask what as it was written in Chinese). At the end of those three treatments, the eczema I had been treating for years was gone! It stayed away for 20 years until I had a small recurrence that I used HEEL'S homeopathic "eczema" formula for. I also found out within the last couple of years that I have an allergy to the whey in dairy and stay away from that now.

What if you are scared of needles altogether? I found a study that shows acupressure is helpful, and for this treatment there are no needles involved! It's called the Tunia technique, and it's a type of massage that stimulates acupressure points, helping healing energy to flow easily. Don't brush this off, the study found that acupressure massage was as good as certain medicines, such as zinc oxide ointment combined with the antihistamine chlorpheniramine.

The research was published in the 2009 issue of *Chinese Medicine and Moxibustion* (Zhongguo Zhen Jiu for all my fans over there). Anyway, the scientists tracked 240 children with eczema, and treated half of them with acupuncture and half with the medicine listed above. 94 to 99% of children receiving Tuina experienced improvement. The kids receiving medicine and ointment achieved a therapeutic benefit in 98 to 100%.

For all practical purposes this is about the same efficacy rate, but here's the shocker. Six months after treatment, the recurrence rate was only 3.8% in the Tuina group but it was 43% in the medication group. So the kids who got the acupressure didn't have as high a relapse rate. Isn't that just amazing?!

It impresses me because moms spend thousands of dollars on expensive medications, and here's a study showing that something as simple as acupressure could have a profound effect, assuming you are one of the lucky ones. The researchers concluded: "Tuina on ten points for treatment of infants' eczema has unequivocal short-term effect, a stable long-term effect, and low recurrence rate."

Chapter 20

What Should You Wear?

This is an interesting question because clothing affects people differently. We express ourselves with our clothing. And of course, we all want to be comfortable and stylish. When it comes to eczema though, it does appear to matter.

If you have eczema, you likely already know that certain fabrics can irritate you. In fact, you probably could have written this section for me! But even though I don't have eczema, I do tend to have sensitive skin, meaning I can try something on in a department store and within 30 seconds I know if I want that fabric on me, or not. My skin will get itchy until I take it off.

For example, I cannot wear cashmere; it makes me itch. So does wool. Where I live in Colorado, it gets cold, sometimes below zero with the wind chill factor. In January, we wear Teflon underwear around here, tee hee hee. Seriously, some people do need heavier fabrics to sleep in or to wear during the day. If you're hypothyroid, you might be cold all the time, and probably wearing more articles of clothing than your friends. The fact is, everyone's skin is a little different. If you're cold all the time, you might really be hypothyroid, or what I term "thyroid sick" in my #1 best-selling book, "Thyroid Healthy, Lose Weight, Look Beautiful & Live the Life You Imagine." See my website or Amazon to snag a copy of this book. People with thyroid disease are more prone to eczema, and unfortunately testing does not pick up the disorder in most cases. I give you secrets to uncover the truth in my book.

Some people with eczema are very sensitive to a chemical used to dye or treat leather, the kind of leather on a purse or your shoes. If you have hand eczema (dyshidrotic) then this could be your problem. Or your leather couch, or leather-wrapped steering wheel or gear shifter. I bet you never knew that!

Fabrics of Choice, Fabrics to Avoid

Synthetic fabrics. Try to minimize or avoid. These are produced from the chemical processing of petroleum.

Wool. Nope, not good either. It's main constituent is keratin, which is the same protein in our very own skin. You'd think wool would be most compatible on our skin, but in fact wool is highly irritating to people with eczema, and increases itching. The more coarse the wool texture, the more itchy you'll be. I have a hat made of wool that my husband Sam bought me at an art festival that I can't wear because it makes my forehead itch like crazy. It's that sensitizing.

Silk. Natural silk is made by the industrious little silkworm! The thread is composed of a protein material called fibroin, and it's glued together by sericin, a sticky substance. It's woven together into the silky fabric we love. I think it's a trial and error thing, because silk is smooth, and doesn't cause friction on the skin. But most silk clothing will be unacceptable to a person with eczema. (Don't worry if you need stitches, the silk for medical use is specially treated to remove sericin so it's hypoallergenic).

I think certain types of silk can be eczema-friendly; again it's a trial and error thing. Special silk clothing, which is specially treated and known to designers as "DermaSilk," can be helpful, versus regular silk or even cotton. A small study published in the *British Journal of Dermatology* randomly assigned 46 children with eczema to wear this special silk or cotton clothing next to their skin. They only allowed the kids to use a moisturizing cream. After one week there was a significant improvement of eczema in the silk group, but no change in the cotton group.

Cotton. The most frequently recommended fabric, it's soft and naturally abundant. That said, it's prone to infestation of fungi and bacteria. Despite this drawback, cotton is still better than synthetic fabric and wool.

Latex gloves. If you find yourself wearing latex gloves while cleaning, painting, or examining your patients, for example, keep in mind that latex can make your skin angry too. It seems to set off individuals who are particularly sensitive.

Nudist anyone? Well I'm kidding around, because I've given you all these fabric choices, yet none of them are 100% perfect because they can all cause friction on the skin, or cause itchiness, or can be contaminated. I think the best thing is to get to the underlying cause of your eczema, and keep a diary so you can trace back and see what is causing the flares. Once you treat yourself for the underlying problem, you can open up your wardrobe a little bit, and include fabrics that are both fashionable and comfortable.

Looking Good with Sensitive Skin

What about makeup? The make-up you put on your skin is critically important. I can't tell you how many people have come to me saying they have rosacea and used Bare Minerals, thinking it was a natural product and were shocked when it made their condition worse. They did not know it, but this company happens to use bismuth oxychloride, which is considered a cheap filler, and it's in their powders. If you look at this ingredient under a microscope, you'll see it's a very jagged particle. Imagine all those little jagged particles on already sensitive skin. No wonder it made their condition worse!

Bismuth oxychloride is considered a heavy mineral (that resembles arsenic) and requires the ongoing buffing mineral makeup companies advise in order to force it into the skin and pores to keep it from sliding off of your face. It's a by-product of the lead and copper processing industry. Seriously. Read the label on your product to see what's in it, especially if you react to it. Also, you can go to Skin Deep and look it up.

I have a better option for you, if you want to smooth your complexion out and use a powder based make up: Honeybee Gardens Pressed Mineral Foundation. Here is a link to Honeybee's website: http://www.honeybeegardens.com/

I asked the owner for a coupon for my readers, and was given one by Honeybee. If you use "PHARM" at checkout, this company will give you free standard shipping.

It is a very gentle formula, which is great for those with sensitive skin. This product is talc free, paraben free, fragrance free, and oil free. And it contains soothing vitamin E and gentle botanical extracts to calm skin. It's such a versatile product because it can be worn over foundation or directly on bare skin to even out skin tone. It also refines the complexion and reduces shine, leaving a natural, silky finish that is never heavy or cakey-looking. You can use the separately sold foundation pan alone, or use it with a refillable eco-friendly compact and help save the planet (less waste in landfills). Also you can apply the powder with a cotton puff or an eco-friendly, cruelty-free kabuki brush.

Mascara Anyone?

It's very common to have eczema attack the eyelids, making it difficult or impossible to comfortably wear mascara. I can recommend two 2 products that might be gentle enough for you. The first one is called Raw Mascara by Earthlab. This is a lash-defining, weightless mascara that enhances your eyelash color. It goes on light as a feather. Do not expect it to plump you up the way conventional chemical-laden mascara does. This is very gentle, non-smudging and non-flaking. They put something in it to make it moisturizing to your lashes. It is paraben-free and also free of preservatives.

The second mascara I recommend is *Honeybee Garden's Natural Mascara.* This is a gentle, silky, lash-defining mascara that is totally weightless yet provides all-day color. The smooth light-as-a-feather base boasts zero clumping due to the absence of clay in the superior lash-conditioning formula. It won't flake or smudge, but perhaps best of all is this botanically-enriched mascara is paraben free, water-resistant, and work-out proof (not water-proof).

I have it myself in Black Magic and love it, but it also comes in Chocolate Truffle brown, and Espresso Black/Brown. I asked the owner of the company for a coupon for my readers, and she granted me one. If you use "PHARM" at checkout, Honeybee will give you free standard shipping. This coupon code will not work on the Vitacost site though, just from Honeybee.

Chapter 21
Do's and Don'ts

Eczema is a symptom of something else; it's the outward manifestation. It's not a disease in and of itself. It's just telling you that you have something bigger going on. Like fatigue, it's not a disease, but it may alert you to the fact that something else going on. Don't let yourself be defined by eczema. You can overcome it! I have faith in you. Be strong, hold on, and keep researching and trying. One day, you'll hit the jackpot, and you'll be able to help others who reach out to you.

Any doctor will tell you that there is no medical cure for eczema. This is because the cause of dry skin and eczema can be varied in different people.

It is very difficult to find a treatment that is going to help everyone who suffers with dry eczema skin. The reason is because the cause varies. Because of this, a lot of people are turning to alternative eczema treatments, and many are finding real benefits as they treat the root cause.

Dos and Don'ts

Don't – Rub moisturizer onto DRY skin.

Do – Apply moisturizer on damp skin. This helps the skin to retain moisture longer. You can moisturize right after your shower/bath, or you can use a gentle spray toner to wet your skin right before applying your lotion. One of my favorite spray toners is Balancing Facial Toner made by Boscia. I spray it on all day long when it gets dry here. Another favorite is Naturopathica's Rose Geranium Soothing Mist, which contains ingredients known to sooth dry itchy, skin. It also contains galactoarabinan, a natural polysaccharide extracted from North America larch trees. It could help with skin tone and fine lines. Keep your skin moist.

You can even make your own facial toners, which I do myself at home. I take distilled water and add lavender, frankincense and myrrh essential oils. I mist my face all day. After you mist your face with your toner of choice, apply your serum and lotion.

Don't – Wear pajamas or clothing made of man-made materials. They contain irritating chemicals. It's okay if you want to be playful and wear something sexy and lacy for a short time. I totally get that, but while you're sleeping, working, or running errands, wear natural and breathable fabric.

Do – Stick to cotton where possible.

Don't – Use lotions or cosmetics which contain alcohol, dyes, or perfumes.

Do – Apply only the most natural ingredients.

Don't – Scratch. I know that's impossible, so just do the best you can. When your skin is dry, it's the most itchy, so keep it nicely moist.

Do – Keep your fingernails short. (Or put gloves on your baby's hands.)

Don't – Wear costume jewelry, especially if you're having a rough month. Same applies to metallic headbands, earrings, bangles, chunky necklaces, belt buckles, and watches, etc.

Do- Accessorize. I'm a bit of a fashionista and would go crazy if I couldn't wear the stuff above. How about I make a deal with you? Give up all those goodies 'til your skin clears, and instead, buy a lovely pair of funky shoes or a bold purse that makes a statement, or try a pretty headband that is made of cloth or even plastic (not metal). Feeling funky? Get a colorful hair extension you can clip in for a few hours, it gives you a strand of color that is sexy and subtle. These options should be safe for you, and still offer a little spark of style, taking your mind off the fact that you can't wear your beloved jewelry. Remember, 18-24K yellow gold may be okay for you. Here's another idea, ask your local jeweler to trade in your 10-14K gold towards something you *can* wear. Gold is at a good price right now too, so your trade in will take you far.

Don't – Allow your skin to get too hot. Central heating, sunlight, and saunas can be a trigger.

Do – Buy a humidifier for your bedroom.

Don't – Allow harsh chemicals or detergents to touch your bare skin when cleaning.

Do – Wear gloves to do household chores or special projects.

Don't – Eat refined sugar or dairy. I think honey and maple syrup, or coconut nectar are all fine. Unrefined blue agave (raw) is okay too.

Do- Wear gloves if you type on keyboards or laptops where your hands touch metal.

Don't – Become too dependent on prescribed steroids or you'll never get to the underlying cause.

Do – Try to uncover the underlying cause. Never give up. Ever.

Do – Consume lots of fresh vegetables and mineral water. You want to achieve a more alkaline state.

Good luck and God speed! I wish you well :-)

To stay in touch with me, sign up to receive my free newsletter, which I send out about once a week. The sign up page is at my website

Bonus Section

Friends Helping Friends

I love to ask others to share their personal stories and Facebook is the perfect place for that. Recently, I asked my fans and friends there to share any tips that helped them personally, or helped a loved one with eczema. Here are some of the best tips that they shared on July 9th, 2012. I'm including these in this book because there is likely something here that can help you. Some of the people referred to products or websites and you may see some of my personal notes or clarifications in between the [brackets] within their comments.

Harmony Health- From my experience, tea tree oil ointments work best. But the idea of watching what you eat when it occurs is good too. Food journaling is a good way to keep track. Usually food allergies stem from wheat, dairy, or citrus. Take a good look at what you eat for breakfast every day. :)

Lori- Our teenage son had horrible, cracked, raw knuckles with eczema this past winter. We used coconut oil every morning and night, covering his hands while he slept, and it cleared up immediately. No problems since. Also did the same for another young son who developed a single spot on a lower leg. It, too, cleared up when an Rx from our doctor did nothing.

Vicky- Low Dose Naltrexone or LDN... definitely look into this for your article! [Here's a website devoted to LDN: www.lowdosenaltrexone.org

Jocelyn- The two biggest offenders are dairy and wheat. Remove them and you see dramatic changes. Homeopathically I use Sulphur for most eczema, but other remedies that are part of the person's overall symptoms picture can be: Pulsatilla, Causticum, Arscenicum, Sepia. There is a mental emotional picture to this as well: stress, anxiety can go right to the skin. Second recommendation of remedies are best for those situations. But as in all holistic health care, everyone is different and is evaluated as such, best remedy for them not a one size fits all.

Jenna-African Black Soap has helped me.

Amy- I suffered for years with eczema, but no longer have problems! I follow a VERY strict gluten free diet! I also do not consume dairy, except for some occasional raw cheese, or goat cheese. I don't eat processed foods either! I prepare every one of my families meals at home. I am thankful to God for the wisdom he gave me.

Kelly- Stay away from sugar, corn, yeast, or anything that contains them.

Amy- I am also a Young Living essential oil distributor, so I use their supplements and oils, and their cleaning products! I don't use chemicals in my home because they cause asthma attacks.

Maria- My daughter had eczema on her legs and arms until age 8. I tried every remedy, every medicated cream etc... Nothing worked as well as Aquaphor healing ointment and Curel original formula. The trick is to apply lotions with wet/damp skin and rub until it dissolve in the affected area. Also used Zyrtec or Claritin for flair up days.

Amy- I make my own herbal lotion, have had great success with eczema. It contains Cedarwood, Bergamot, Ginger, Orange, Peppermint and Tea Tree, all in a beeswax base with olive, grape seed, and jojoba. Of course, that is just a topical treatment. Also have used yucca root internally as a blood cleanser and had success with clearing up chronic eczema outbreaks. That, and I only use lye soap on the skin, no perfumes or detergents. :)

Mimi- I take pharmaceutical grade fish oil for eczema.

Carina- Aloe vera is the only thing that works on my eczema, either straight from the plant or a cream... it is amazing stuff!

Renee- Low Dose Naltrexone (LDN) works to modulate the immune system, therefore no more skin issues!! I use if for Fibro. I you want to learn more, message me and I will send you a request to join my LDN group on facebook so you can learn more, or just google LDN and any auto immune issues for a great surprise!!

Karen- I have scalp psoriasis, and homeopathic sulphur 30x works as well as local cortisone injections.

Carol- I had eczema for years and still get small outbreaks on my hands in the winter, but I can't get over how much improvement I've had since changing my diet to an alkaline one. In addition to that, I started seeing a chiropractor, and I know that has had a great impact. Using extra-virgin coconut oil on my skin has been very helpful also.

Mike- With my nephew we and doctors thought he had ring worm, as it was showing up in small dots with a clear center resembling ring worm. So we used anti-fungal (athletes foot) creams and a steroid lotion (forgot name of it). It wasn't until he had a big outbreak on his butt, then did the doctor say he had eczema. So we treat by giving occasional oatmeal bathes and eczema creams (NOT LOTIONS), and I still use the anti-fungal creams too because that seems to work much faster. Keep the skin well creamed will help keep outbreaks at bay!

Shane- My last flare up was from drinking beer. I broke out in hives, blisters, eczema, contact dermatitis, psoriasis, and was so swollen with arthritis flares that I could not open my hands. My temperature was 106. I saw 7 doctors in ONE day at the hospital and even 2 heads of departments that are university researchers were at a loss how to treat this. I left with $700 in topical creams, none of which were effective! My general practitioner saw me a few days later and ordered a juice fast...desperate for relief I tried it and it worked. My blood work showed massive immune responses and I was placed on low-dose naltrexone (LDN) for a month. My doctor said "You are just hours away from permanent arthritis, all it takes is just ONE cell to confuse undigested proteins in your blood stream with joint tissues and you will never walk again." A hard dose of reality! In 3 days of fasting and the LDN, everything subsided and I started a regime probiotics. I have not (thankfully) had another flare up/attack. I was under the impression that it was the gluten in beer but perhaps it was the hops? I'm not certain but I avoid bread generally but on occasion eat it but I have not touched beer in 15 months!

Donna- Probiotics!!!!

Jim- A former client of mine claims that AcneStatin works wonders.

Inabathini- Though, I haven't faced any skin problems, I heard 'E45' cream from England works great on eczema. Worth trying, folks!

Joan- White vinegar

Mary- Gluten-free diet

Teena- CeraVe Moisturizing Cream (not lotion). It has helped my father-in-law tremendously!
It contains no fragrance to irritate the skin, but it does contain ceramides. These are natural fatty compounds found in cell membranes. People with eczema frequently have lower levels of ceramides in their skin.

Doug- Eliminating food sensitivities (IgA, IgG, IgE) is a must. Solvent exposures need to be eliminated from the home.

Gurdip- Tea Tree Oil and plenty of fluids (preferably water)! [Tea tree oil is sold at many pharmacies, but usually at health food stores and many online retailers]

Shirley- Coconut oil helps

Seloa- change of lifestyle and get a food allergy test. It worked for me. Haven't had it for 2 years now!!!

Nikole- I have psoriasis, I have had it as long as I can remember and tried hundreds of different treatments, diets, creams, lotions, masks, you name it. So far the best thing I have been given by my doctor to try is Desitin cream. I think it has to do with the Zinc since other products that I have tried with Zinc seem to help a wee bit. The runner up as far as what has worked best for me is Desonide Cream 0.05%. [Desonide Cream requires a prescription. Desitin is sold at any pharmacy or discount retail store like Target/Walmart.]

Hillary- Mine was so bad, down my neck, behind my ears... I even had hair loss. As a teenager, I would pour Pro-Topic on my head, nothing would work! But, my symptoms would go away in the summer. Come to find out, it was because my grandparents had a pool, and I was always in it. So, swimming in a pool works for me. Completely clears it up! I am not sure if it is the chlorine or what... but, as long as I swim 2-3 times a week I am E- Free! And medication free too!

Perla- Cetaphil cream really worked for my family! And at the same time keeping the skin clean and w/o toxins and perfumes....

Morag- Terra-Cortril Ointment is very good for face eczema. [This is a prescription salve that is based on a tetracycline type of antimicrobial called "oxytetracycline." Terra-Cortril is available as an eye drop.]

James- Ok, I don't know if anyone else tried this just for eczema but since I was over 65 my general practitioner suggested I get the shot for Shingles, and so I did. Eczema is totally different. but after the shot my arm was really sore for about a month, like a bad reaction. However, my eczema was quite suppressed after that ordeal. Like all the people who get eczema I've tried not eating things I thought might cause it. I found that mentally focusing on eczema with

"Intention" and similar modalities in that arena I helped it much better than strange diets and lotions. Doctors I've seen had only general products for this specific problem. Right now I'm wondering if I increase my iodine or iodide if that may help. Another supplement that interests me is L-cysteine and Alpha Lipoic Acid. Eczema is triggered by certain stress issues. Finding the switch to turn off chronic flares is a game plan. There are around 30 or so modalities along with Acupuncture that have been of use or some people.

Mary- My daughter owns a company called January Labs. She has a cleanser that is awesome and seems to cure a eczema break out...it is her Skin Essentials pure and gentle cleansing gel....it has willow bark in it which is awesome.... hope that helps.

Darla- As soon as I cut out gluten, my eczema went away. I also improved my diet by cutting out concentrated sweets and floury carbs, ate lots more fresh greens.

Ruth- For my eczema problem I got some help from cactus juice products--all day energy greens and that pink bottle stuff they advertise on tv--the all day energy greens were the cheapest way to go--almost half the cost of the other stuff--it helped my rosacea too some--I also believe it is, as the Eastern culture calls it, a Hot disorder that needs cooling with alkaline veggies and inflammation Sonoma cactus concoctions. When I eat more greens and more fruits and less of the wheat carbs I find it is less. Taking the green stuff reduced it by almost 80%, and that's a lot. It isn't as flared up as it was. I also think drinking plenty of water helps the skin a lot. I also use the Q1000 laser on it as well to help heal areas that get scraped looking. I also think that EFT* helps to to quell the anxiousness of spirit that creates acid in our bodies. It's a healing technique used to treat PTSD (post-traumatic stress disorder) in veterans, and firemen and police departments. It also can be used as a healing meditation while tapping on acupressure meridians. When you use this technique you get a physical sigh release and feel less overwhelmed about things. A nurse did a test on clumpy blood cells on a person with low energy. After using EFT her cells were not clumpy and were moving better. A lot of this info is on youtube. [*EFT means Emotional Freedom Technique. Find information here: *www.thetappingsolution.com*]

Chaz- An anti-fungal diet will help! Try oil of oregano topically for this problem.

Denise- Coconut oil is excellent for psoriasis and skin problems.

Marisa- My 3-year-old daughter has eczema, and we have cut out (for the most part) gluten and dairy. We also use red clover plus salve on her patches, which has worked very well. We make sure she is rinsed thoroughly after being in a chlorinated pool and that she is dried well and quickly after bathing.

Andrea- 2 ounces of unpasteurized butter a day. Heard this at an IFHI conference [Institute for Human Individuality]. Following the blood type diet. It is always about what you do eat that heals.

Chantell- For my son I used avocado oil with rose, geranium, chamomile, and frankincense essential oils.

Eddie- Peel a plantain, inside part of the peel, when you work with plantain you cannot touch a white shirt, due to the acid on it will turn it black permanently. This acid rubbed on face seems to kill facial infections, old Puerto Rican remedy.

Ros- Honey mask draws out toxins.

Julie- I had a customer who had it very bad. She did bio-feedback and got off of
the foods she was sensitive and allergic to, and it all cleared up.

Pam- Wheat was my problem.

Georgia- My husband has eczema, but it is minor to what he had. The doctors gave him all kinds of meds that did not work and cost a fortune. He now uses Extra Virgin olive oil. He puts in his bath water and then on his skin afterwards. It's the only thing that has worked for him. I would say it decreased it by 90%.

Priscilla- ARGAN oil. Nothing else needed. Anytime my son has a flare up I treat
it and it subsides.

Annie- For many years I have been plagued with eczema. For relief, I used OTC 1% Hydrocortisone Anti-Itch Cream. That was effective, but certainly not a cure. I also covered my body with Cetaphil (best for me) lotion after a shower. A few months ago, I came across a publication about synthetic cosmetic ingredients to avoid. I decided to give that a try. I mostly did away with phthalates, parabens, and petrochemicals. I started eliminating lipstick then purchasing the chemical free products for my hair and face care. The results have been amazing. It has been months, and I have not had one eczema flare up. Such a relief! I tried various herbs to no avail. This has worked for me.

Joyce- Raw apple cider vinegar with the mother in it is good. Antifungals are a must, and change the diet, and stay away from sugar and sugar foods. Minerals to support the body, vitamin A. Also, baking soda and Epsom salts are good for the skin. Be blessed.

Sara- My 10-year-old son has battled this for about 18 months now. We are having huge success now. He is almost clear, and he has an extreme case. Noticed the biggest jump in healing when we started with digestive enzymes. (We took him off gluten, dairy, and a host of other foods about 7 months ago) The next jump in healing seems to have coincided with BioResonance therapy. We are starting to re-introduce mozzarella cheese, mild cheddar, and a few other things with no reaction. We'll see what the winter weather brings.

Gerry- About 20 years ago, I used Astragalus Tabs. Itching went away in one day
and skin cleared in about 3 days. Problem never returned.

Karen- This is a yeast overgrowth condition. Lots of probiotics and a yeast fighter like Florastor would be a good idea.

Angela- Eliminate foods you are intolerant to. Works for my little one.

Lori- When I was in high school my Aunt Hazel went to the drug store and got powdered sulfur (yellow) and we mixed it with Vasoline. It worked when nothing else would. Almost overnight. I don't know if powdered sulfur is available now at the pharmacy, but if it is, try it.

John- Coconut oil, worked for me.

Alicia- Colloidal Silver Gel and coconut oil. Cleared up and completely in 3 days

Anna- I had a very good experience with using Ganoderma Lucidum soap, is 100% natural product.

Eva- Sea buckthorn oil!!! Works on eczema as well as rosecea!

Mary- Have you seen the movie Fat Sick and Tired? He lost his eczema in a month by only drinking fresh juices.

Sharon- Silver Solution: Antifungal, Antibacterial, and AntiviralDiane- Sunshine works best for me

Christopher- First, cut out dairy and grains, add zinc and natural vitamin A

Sally- The white side of potato skin. apply securely, bandage, leave overnight

Connie- Raleigh's salve is the best I can recommend...works for all ages Diane- Swimming in a salt-filtered pool and the eczema healed in two days of swimming.

Connie- My grandmother always swore by washing the area with pine tar soap. It smells bad but she said it always worked for her.

Live the Healthy Edge- Take fish oil and evening primrose oil, remove all food allergens

Appendix 1- List of Topical Steroids

These medications require prescriptions unless otherwise specified:

Seriously potent

- Betamethasone dipropionate 0.05% (Diprolene)
- Clobetasol propionate 0.05% (Dermovate)
- Halobetasol propionate (Ultravate)
- Halcinonide 0.1% (Halog)

Potent:

- Amcinonide 0.1% (Cyclocort)
- Betamethasone dipropionate 0.05% (Diprosone, generics)
- Betamethasone valerate 0.05% (Betaderm, Celestoderm, Prevex)
- Desoximetasone 0.25% (Desoxi, Topicort)
- Diflucortolone valerate 0.1% (Nerisone)
- Fluocinonlone acetonide 0.25% (Fluoderm, Synalar)
- Fluocinonide 0.05% (Lidemol, Lidex, Lyderm, Tiamol, Topsyn)
- Fluticasone propionate (Cutivate)

- Halcinonide (Halog)
- Mometasone furoate 0.1% (Elocom)

Moderately potent:

- Betamethasone valerate (Betnovate, Betaderm, Celestoderm)
- Clobetasone butyrate 0.05% (Eumovate or Trimovate)
- Hydrocortisone acetate 1.0% (Cortef, Hyderm)
- Hydrocortisone valerate 0.2% (Westcort, HydroVal)
- Prednicarbate 0.1% (Dermatop)
- Triamcinolone acetonide 0.1% (Kenalog, Triaderm)

Mild action:

- Desonide 0.05% (Desocort)
- Hydrocortisone 2.5% (Cortate, Cortisone, Cortoderm)
- Hydrocortisone acetate 0.5 - 1% (Hyderm)
- Hydrocortisone 0.5 - 1% (Cortaid, Cortisone) These strengths do not require prescription.

CPSIA information can be obtained
at www.ICGtesting.com
Printed in the USA
LVOW01s0629300916
506592LV00003B/389/P

9 781505 529029